Secrets of Longevity ... Revealed

Live from 100 to 200 years

____

By Grand master M. Jayanth Reddy
Winner of 29 Guinness World Records

ISBN 9781686006784

Printed in USA by Print on Demand with Amazon.

Dedication

This book is dedicated to my mother Late. Smt. Morramganti Shivamma and my father Late Sri. Morramganti Vithal Reddy.

Phone: 91-9391007598

Email: mjayanthreddy03@gmail.com

Table Of Contents

Foreword

"Knowing is not enough, one has to experience the beauty of the universe" – M. Jayanth Reddy

May this book bring you the in-depth information about our living, how we are, the balance between the human and the universe, the energy and life of you and worldly people in this planet earth. Its already inbuilt by God within yourself all the possibilities – and only you should have capacity to believe or experience it. One can search on internet for the definition of fitness, written by multiple sources – amateur to expert. There are also innumerable books on fitness and life. My honest view is that all knowledge read is of no use; one must experience. Once you experience the beauty of the universe, you will realize that the universe is for the living beings and the most exciting time is to experience the history of the humans, the cycle of life, how impossible becomes possible – a study in every field of human endeavor in health and life of this magnificence of the human kind.

My whole intention of writing this book is for the wellbeing of mankind and the entire world.

Phone: 91-9391007598

Email: mjayanthreddy03@gmail.com

Preface

In this book, I have mentioned simple exercises, physical, breathing techniques and healing sounds. Learn, experience and appreciate these – and appreciate yourself. See all that - without judgement and then appreciate the long path of learning that led you to this point in life, appreciate the effort you put into surviving and learning the ancient medicinal exercises. I have sacrificed much for this information. See all of it, see it without judgement but with clarity and then advice everyone to take to themselves. Nobody in this world helps you; and this world has become most egoistic and selfish. Further no one helps you in anyway. And so, this is my healthy wish to you to help yourself. If you die, is there anyone coming with you? No one. You are only one who can be yourself. Your family, your relations, your business is attached externally, and it detaches from you, the moment you leave the house (planet earth). My point is, experience my exercise. If you feel good, continue – else leave this. I am not going to retaliate to your facial expression or emotional reaction. I have good sense to develop humans to the ultimate being of longevity on the planet earth.

This book is like unshaped rock in your hands to design yourself. You can make greatest sculptor or a monument of ancient world or a famous personality. You can be one of them only if you cut into the shape with patience. You can reach it!!

I wish that for you!

Introduction

"Human body is the living book" – M. Jayanth Reddy

The health of human being is placed in such floods and over pouring science the past two centuries. We seem to find ourselves in a far-off shallow. When this world awakes, people of this modern world will all realize that the progress in science and technology has brought on us a common injury in the form of imbalances of nature. Chemical foods, fast foods and pollution of the atmosphere, stress, egos, and worries have imperiled our human lives. No scientist nor any leader nor spiritual person any religious person is helping the humanity to get rid of these. Life science should be the ideal tool which blends all universal secrets for ultimate health and longevity. The universal secrets range from ancient breathing techniques to atmospheric engineering that can assist our present health and healing, thereby increasing the quality of this universe which will in turn have a positive effect on our goal of healing, well-being and longevity.

As we all very well know, present day medical treatment seems inadequate for our sufferings caused by the modern day. There is a lurking danger in our health, which is not only hidden from us but which even doctors are failing to identify perfectly to heal permanently. It is affecting nearly almost every one of us – no matter how active or sedentary you are, how old or young you are, this problem affects not only our body but our whole well-being.

We are fast approaching the 21st century and mankind is praying for peace and health in all nook and corners of this world. Now we must come in a single platform to deal with it and we must help each other in this life. There is no other way but to cooperate and collaborate. We need to teach our younger generation and learn from those who have knowledge and experience of health and peace. We are all one – though we are from different religions, regions, countries and continents – we are humans. God made kingdom of humans, animals and spices etc. on this same say. We must understand this fact and realize the truth that we all must think unitedly for universal health.

Remember – "Human body is the living book; all other written books are spoken words only". That way all books are which are written by many people in this world are useless, until we open our own book.

Today's world

"What a disgrace it is for a man to grow old without ever seeing the beauty and strength of which his body is capable". M. Jayanth Reddy

Human body is made to live up to 1000 Years, but we are not living for at least 100 Years in the 21st Century.

The problem:

The Problems of youth is a major concern for parents, schools, religious institutions and social agencies as much in our country and as well across the globe. These problems are reflected in part by much of anti-social behavior that has captured the headlines in the international and nation's electronic and print media during the past few years. The entire world is concerned about things such as - student activism leading to violence, the use of Cigarettes, alcohol, drugs and narcotics, the increase in number of rape's, unwed mothers', divorces and poor health of many young people.

Root cause:

Dr. Robert Milliken, a Nobel Prize winner in science, has said that "the age of invention has brought the age of discovery - the age of discovery has brought the age of power and the age of power has brought the age of leisure".

As Charles A. Bucher, an eminent physical educationist, has pointed out that throughout the world man appears to be living a more and more inactive/sedentary life, he rides instead of walking, sits instead of standing and watches instead of participating.

Advancement of science and technology replaced manual labor with machines and gadgets, thus creating lot of leisure time – resulting in tension and stress related diseases.

Late. John Edger Hoover a Director of Federal Bureau of Investigations of USA said that he has booked many of the country's youth between 12 to 18 years of age and that the crime by them was increasing day by day because of abundant leisure. He says that youth is responsible for 7.4 million automobile thefts, 15.8 burglaries, 2.7 million robberies, 3 million assaults, 2.3 million murders, bank hold ups and other crimes. India also is topping the list of crime by youth in the age of 16 to 25 years – rape, drugs and anti-social behaviors.

John Edger hoover analyzed the causes of crimes and listed them as follows. Youth involve in criminal and anti-social activities primarily listed below.

"As such criminals are made not born", he concludes.

Mayour Morrison feels that if the kids could blow off their excess steam and energy in the field, they would not blow safes in the banks. The kids who steal bananas from the next house should be stealing second base in softball game.

The leading Killers of mankind in the early part of this century were Obesity, diabetes, Cancer, Kidney failure, lungs deficiencies, mental disease, and Blood pressure, Pneumonia, Influenza, Tuberculosis, Diarrhea, Enteritis, Intestinal Ulcers, Heart Diseases, Cerebral Hemorrhage and Nephritis. Today, however, the order has changed to some extent. Diseases of the heart now lead the list with such maladies as Cancer, Intra Cranial Lesions of Vascular region, Nephritis. Pneumonia, etc.

It can be seen from these listings that infectious diseases are being brought under control by the medical profession. However, diseases which are concerned with the heart, blood vessels, and kidneys have rushed to the front and it is difficult to bring them under control. Some experts believe that these deaths are largely due to the tensions and stress of modern life.

Howard Whitman showed how cases of Heart diseases fluctuated with the fortunes of the stock market. How many top executives in business were paid large salaries but killed themselves to break production records? How heart rates increased through emotional tension and how coronary diseases were twice as prevalent among people doing sedentary work, as among those who were active in their jobs. He stated that to have a healthy life a man should not lead a highly competitive existence and try not to be a money slave. Rather, he must enjoy life with his family and neighbors and learn to play and enjoy day to day living.

P.M. John, in his best seller, "Point of No. return", shows how man is continually striving to get ahead in his work, and in so doing, how he burns himself out and in the end is left bereft of all spiritual props which alone make life worthwhile.

People should understand that one can't buy health with money….and that one can't take his property with him when he dies. If one is not healthy, he will live shorter and die longer.

He continually wants a bigger car, a more luxurious home, and a more elite school for his Children, nice clothes and desires to belong to a more fashionable country club. In striving for all these things, however, he constantly experiences tension and does not enjoy the things that make life worthwhile. Finally, he reaches the point of no-return, the point at which he doesn't have an option of turning back and he must go on living this unbearable existence to the end.

Solution:

Swami Vivekananda quoted "You Will Be Nearer to Heaven through Football than through the Study of the Gita"- emphasizing the need of physical health and its influence on sound mind.

This is where physical education can take over. Physical education activities may contribute considerably in relieving the tension of modern day living. When an individual is attempting to break part sport activities or when he is attempting to serve a tennis "ACE", he forgets all about the conference with the boss the next day, about the final examination in English, or about getting a higher salary and a better job to that of door neighbor. The tension that has gripped his body all day is finally relieved through his interest and enthusiasm for this wholesome activity.

Since many youth and adults do not fully understand and appreciate the importance of health and fitness, great responsibility rests on the shoulders of educators. If an action is to remain strong physically, mentally, spirituality and socially, there must be education for fitness.

Furthermore, this education must take place largely through the formal process of physical education, health education and recreation programs in schools, colleges, institutions and various firms. Knowledge about the human body must be imparted, desirable health attitudes inculcated, and proper health practices instilled. The responsibility for accomplishing this herculean task must be assumed mainly by physical educators, health educators and recreation educators, and they must continually strive for sound school and community program in their special fields.

According to many health experts, the way each human being lives will be a major determining factor for the health and fitness of that individual. Although heredity plays a part to a large degree, health and fitness are essential characteristics of healthy individuals. The Food that is eaten, amount of rest taken, physical activity engaged in and other health practices that are followed play important roles in determining human welfare. In other words, it is important to follow a good health regimen if one is to be healthy, fit and continue to be at ease from various diseases.

Former US President Kennedy stated that "the strength of our democracy is no greater than the collective wellbeing of our people". The vigor of our country is no stranger than the vitality and will of our countrymen. The level of physical mental, moral and spiritual fitness of every Individual in Indian and aboard must be our constant concern.

Physical Fitness:

"We do not stop exercising because we grow old – we grow old because we stop exercising."

As such fitness is the ability of a person to live a full and balanced existence. The totally fit person not only possess physical wellbeing but also have qualities such as good human relations, maturity and high ethical standards of our modern civil society. He or she also satisfies the basic needs as love, affection, security and self-respect.

The term physical fitness implies soundness of internal body organs (heart, kidneys, liver, stomach and lungs, a human mechanism and circulation system) performed efficiently under exercise or work conditions, such as having enough stamina and strength to engage in vigorous physical activity and a reasonable measure of skill in the performance of selected physical activities.

The physical fitness plan of a person must be done in relation to a person's own human resources and not those of others. It depends on one's potentialities in the light of individual physical make up. Finally, physical fitness cannot be considered by itself but, instead as it is affected by mental, emotional and social factors as well. Human beings' function and not as segmented points.

1.   Physically fitness required regular medical examinations

2.   You are what you eat, the right kind of food should be eaten in the right amounts.

3.   Exercise is important as such select the physical activities according to the age.

4.   Adequate sleep, rest and relaxation is a must for 6 to 8 hours.

Norms of physical fitness for the noncompetitive persons:

Types of Exercise:
There are four types of exercises which are listed in the below picture.

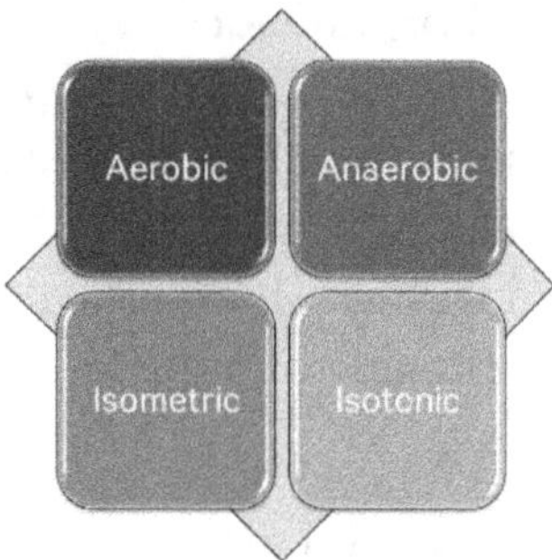

Will focus on Aerobic exercise, which is key for physical fitness

More and more people are accepting the fact that aerobic exercise is essential to a healthy cardiovascular system. In brief aerobic exercise is an activity that can be sustained for an extended period without building an oxygen debt in the muscles. It is a type of exercise that overloads the heart and lungs and causes them to work harder than they do when a person is at rest. Aerobic exercise typically engaging in activities such as jogging, skipping, bicycling, swimming and walking.

Some of the benefits of aerobic exercise includes the ability to utilize more oxygen during strenuous exercise a lower heart rate at rest, the production of less lactic acids and greater endurance. Also, many exercise physiologists have found that it reduces blood pressure and changes blood chemistry. It also improves the efficiency of the heart, more evidence is needed to substantiate the belief by some persons that aerobic exercise is responsible for the development of supplemental blood vessels to the heart, which would be helpful in the event of a heart attack and also that such exercise results in increasing the size of coronary arteries and assisting the flow of blood to the heart when the artery is narrowed by clot or arthrosclerosis.

Before a person engages in strenuous exercise, it is recommended that a physician's approval or in any instances a stress test be taken those persons who are approved for activity should plan a progressive program. Starting slowly and gradually increasing the intensity of the exercise until they reach an exercise level that conditions their heart.

Aerobic exercise is for noncompetitive persons who are engaged in sedentary type of work.

Jogging:
In recent years, jogging, which is basically a combination of walking and running has become popular as an aid to keeping physically fit. It has received wide approval from many groups because it is a sustained type of expertise that is noncompetitive. An individual does not have to possess any skill to jog, and most of the joggers' range in age from 35 to 65 years can learn to jog at a good pace. It is extremely important for individuals to have a medical examination or a stress test and to discover the limits of their hearts endurance however before beginning to jog. Jogging has been found beneficial to some heart. It increases the flow of blood to the damaged heart and it may also help some heart attack victims to rebuild the endurance in their heart and lungs. Studies proved that exercise such as jogging force the body to become conditioned to an increased need for oxygen there by strengthening the cardiopulmonary and oxygen transport systems. Among other benefits, jogging also helps in losing weight and frees from stress.

Benefits for mental health
The benefits to sound mental health are especially great when a person engages in games and aerobic activities. One finds great release from tensions, forgets troubles and feels calm. Dr. William Menninger the famous psychiatrist, pointed out that physical activity provides an outlet for instructive, aggressive drives by enabling an individual to "blow off steam", provides relaxation and is a supplement for daily work. He stressed the fact that recreation, which is literally re-creating relaxation from regular activity, is a morale builder - it is not luxury, a waste of time, or a sin.

Although exercise has many physical mental and social benefits, this does not mean a person should rush out and buy a tennis racket and schedule there sets of tennis for Saturday afternoon. To secure these benefits, one must exercise with discretion. Following are some suggestions that reflect the opinion of medical experts and provide good advice for physical educations:

1. Encourage a thorough medical examination at regular intervals to determine the type of exercise most beneficial to the individual.

2. Encourage people to select, if possible, a sport or an activity around the house, such as gardening, cycling, skipping in preference to calisthenics, the mental and social values are greater.

3. After 40 years of age encourage people to cut down on the explosive sports requiring fast starts, and prolonged activity without rest.

4. if a person is out of training in a sport, advise him or her to return to action gradually a little today and a little more tomorrow is a good prescription.

5. Encourage persons to exercise out of doors if possible.

6. Encourage person to select activities that are adopted to them.

7. Encourage people to give their full attention to the activity and have good feelings at the office.

8. Encourage individuals engaging in sports that not to involve body contact or martial arts to use essential protective equipment, especially for head, neck, eyes, teeth, chest, stomach and groin.

9. Encourage individuals to play in areas where safety precautions have been taken to avoid the danger of injuries.

10. Encourage individuals to participate with other of the approximate same degree of skill.

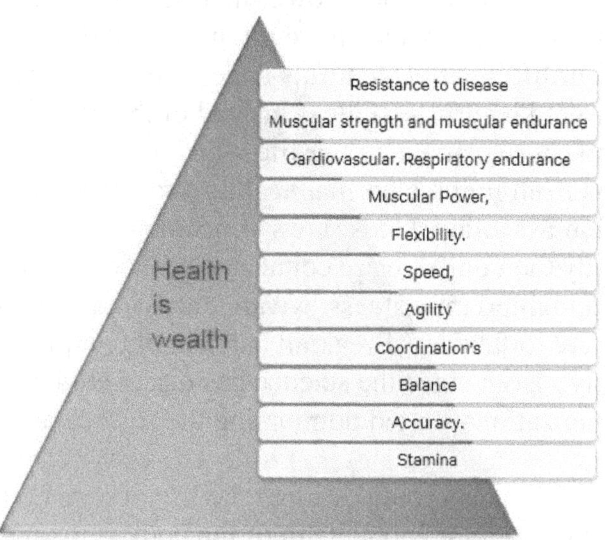

Key Benefits

Body is the God's gift
"Life is God's gift; and what you do with that life is your gift to God"

Your body is directly connected to God. He made you the system of multi organ function with energy the moment you were born.

Today's world is not understanding the mechanism of Human Body, man is compromising the quality of life with poor care of his body. Many even attract diseases.

When we were born, the body was powered by pure body energy and not the mind. We possessed the feeling of our true self when we are our won true self (body feelings), we feel we are complete being inside and that we are naturally connected to the entire outside world. We have the authentic feeling that we are the center of the world, even if we know nothing of the world; we have no worries, neither do we fear anything for us nor do we fear anything, for we are a true part of the entire world in an authentic way. We already know everything that we need to know. This is the gift of God.

While we are growing up, we are introduced to a vast network of artificial symbols and manmade rules, because we were trained to respond to mental concepts, we no longer depend on our feelings of body or to communicate to sunrise. We traded our feeling of life energy and its vast resources with pollution, which consumes and finally burns goal of body's life. The process of depleting and weakening the body functions even though we are completely unaware of it while we are growing up caused our body into diseases, similarly our feeling of us true identify includes our symbolic name and our artificial sense of responsibility. This indicates even further damage to the quality and integrity of our life of God given gift. The more unnatural we become, we pay the price of not following our true life, ignoring and retarding our true body. Our experience of approval for being or looking nice turns out to be very short life span event.

The wealthier and more successful we are, which is judged by artificial rules made by artificial others, the more we work and relentlessly take risks throughout our life. Consequently, as a price for our quest for wealth and success by chasing our artificial goal even after we become richer and successful, honor, power in artificial world. Worst of all is we are willingly lured into such a busy life that we have no time – not even a second. We later weaken body and weaken our life span. Under this false feeling of life and even don't feel happy. When our life is powered by artificial ideas instead of the true feeling of wellbeing it draws, consumes, exhausts and cause damage to our life which means weak physical and mental condition that presents us from living a normal healthy and peaceful life. People who want to live a real and better life must follow Gods' laws – meaning you must exercise/sweat out or clean every part of the body then only we are connected to God instead of by artificial concepts. As we bind our body and mind into fitness, we are one with the entire world and we should lock all the man-made glare to fake us. Break all barriers of complicated and artificial components of our human society. Even since the science has discovered the functions of body, religious and political organizations started dominating the science and laws of human body.

All the modern treasury of humans is temporary to the life of own body; once you lost the body – all treasure is waste. So, keeping good health of the body is the responsibility of every human being. God always wants us to be disease free; we only lost our contact with God because of this so called modern civilized human society.

God always connects with planets and its entire nature- we are forgetting his wish and his ultimate goal to make human "to live better life than the animals". So please do follow his wish. Furthermore, he already designed and built the system within each human being to have a connection with entire cosmos and he keeps monitoring – Hence be positive and genuinely do the exercise to clean your body system, thereby connect to the cosmos. Open the doors of your life and enjoy the wonders that await you. David Bohm has written – 'the energy flow can be influenced not only what is happening in and around the body, but even by the sun, Moon and forces from other planets. There is a deep interrelation with human body and nature.

Further I must mention that in this book I am not mentioning the details about Physiology or anatomy of the human body rather I mention the details about proper functions and exercising. "Ever easing and never dis-easing, the secret of human spirit and function of various organs in balance, the God created human body, the ever longest, fabulous year lined on planet earth in human being, we all must thank God who created us".

To appease others, we are constantly improving our appearance through changing our style of clothing, our house our bike/car our career or at times, even surgically altering our body. This is primarily to look good or give a feel good to others.

Without a healthy state of life energy like that of a newborn baby, we feel there are always cavities in our life. We are off-balanced and disabled without a clue of what is going on, and we develop a false feeling that in order to be our true self or even just to maintain temporary balance and comfort we need support and constant help from sources outside of our self. Since we lost contact with our life energy, we no longer have a natural peaceful feeling inside of our self; instead we become restless. We feel there is constantly something wrong or less than perfect about us. We feel we must look for something even though we don't know what or why. We lessen our self-confidence and eventually we have no self-dignity left within us. Without the integrity and balance of our original life energy, life feels like a disaster an endless saga of suffering with many modern diseases.

When we learn the proper way to rebuild our original life energy exercise, we can gradually restore the fully life strength and well-being. With balance of life energy, we will then be able to feel as if we were a newborn baby again. As it is our original life itself and is a wholesome and complete entity which is self-sustainable and needs no extra help. We feel self-confident and poses a sense of natural dignity furthermore we can get rid of our false identify and bring back the feeling of our true self and the true identify granted to us when we were born and given to us by the name of God.

When our life is powered by artificial ideas instead of the true feeling of our life energy, its draws, consumes, exhausts and causes damage to our life energy - which leads to life energy decline and weak life energy; meaning a weak physical and mental condition that prevents us from living normal, healthy and peaceful life. People who want to live a real healthy and better life must first learn how to rebuild and restore their life energy by my secret exercise of Chi and ancient exercises and they can rapidly a totally change - with improved health psychologically and physiologically fit.

Physical Body vs Mind
"Physical body is more knowledgeable than mind" – M. Jayanth Reddy

Human body is a big Universe in itself. It knows what to accept and what not to accept. It knows what is good and what is bad for the body. Body's chemistry including organs know every food of the world. Human body continuously improves itself and fights several hundreds of diseases there by keeping you safe. We the so called modern civilized people, filling every day with unwanted stuff to the body. Even if we stuff and spoil, but still body goes on protecting you.

Body knows what/which proteins, minerals, vitamins and food are good to internal bone health, joint health and various organs within the body, including circulatory system. This human body is a miniature universe. If you see it from the inside – it is so vast, millions and millions of cells and each cell alive with its own life and each cell functioning in such an intelligent manner that it seems almost incredible, impossible and unbelievable. You eat food and the body transforms it into blood, bones and bone marrow. How marvelous it is.

Today's modern medical science only knows not even 10% of the body. If you looked at it from within in, it is a Universe in itself. I have already mentioned it is a miniature universe. If you see it from inside, it's a vast million and trillions of cells and each cell is alive with its own life and each cell functioning in such a careful manner that it seems almost incredible, impossible, and unbelievable. A miracle is happening every moment and each cell functions so systematically in such an orderly way with such an inner discipline that it seems almost impossible. There are almost 70 million cells in our single body with 70 million souls each cell has its own life/soul. These are continuously healing /defending and works for the betterment of our life – whereas the mind is not like body. Body acts immediately if we put anything in the stomach. It can change the attitude of mind. For example - if you take alcohol, what happens to your mind? Alcohol is taken in the body and not in the mind – but what happens to the mind? If you take LSD or any drugs it goes into the body not into the mind, but what happens to the mind? Or if you go on fast, fasting is done by the body, but what happens to the mind? Or from the other end? Mind must be programed/trained. Otherwise it's of no use.

Body without forgetting its functions, unites all organs – including all internal functionaries, if mind takes the body's work - Imagine for a moment what will happen? Man will have to die at early stage because it may forget to digest food or water or any food product. There would be no possibility of your continuing to live because you can forget to breathe when you sleep at night or could forget to make your heartbeat. How would you remember? There are seventy to seventy-five millions of cells working by themselves without any outside influence - even the mind. Further it supports you in every minute of your life – if you love someone – the body supports you; if you want to kill somebody – the body supports you; if you want to protect somebody – the body supports you; The body is your friend and not your enemy - listen to its language. And the body must be taken care of. One should not be against it. If you condemn it, you have already condemned the God.

Every physician should understand the root cause of his patient's problem and not the symptoms or effect. For example, headache or migraine can be treated but if you don't look deep inside as to why the patient has the migraine or headache problem keeps coming back. May be the patient is too burdened, worried/depressed and many more family or societal problems are affecting him/her. Every physician should study the case history of individual patient. Physician may have a license to practice medicine, he may have doctor degree – if he forces the symptoms to disappear through poisons and medicines, and they may disappear for the time being only because the root cause has not been touched at all.
Further it is ridiculous that the disease may be in the feet, but the medicine goes from head to feet. Recess of the body God resides. God has chosen this house of the body to live in. Respect your body, love your body, care about your body, and clean the body by sweating it every day.

Body has many secrets - and it reveals them when it is purified. That's how greatest yogic, Tao and many monks performed extraordinary powers of the body – walked on water and even travelled in air. But modern medical science is based on the dead bodies and their dissections – which is something fundamentally wrong. It has not yet been able to know the living body. To dissect a dead body is one thing, to know something about it is another thing. But to know something about a living body is totally different. Modern science has no way of knowing about the living body. The only way it knows is to butcher it, to cut it, open it – but the moment you cut it, it's no longer the same phenomenon. To understand the flower on the stem on the tree is one thing; to cut it and dissect it is totally another. It is no longer the same phenomenon. Its quality is different.

Albert Einstein the man has some qualities which the corpse will not have and cannot have. A poet dies – the body is there but where is the poetry? A genius dies- the body is there but where is the genius? The body of the idiot and the genius are the same – you will not be able to know by dissecting the body whether it belonged to a genius or an idiot. Whether it belonged to a mystic or to someone who was never aware of anything mysterious in life. It will be impossible because you are simply looking into the house and the being who lived there is no more there. You are simply studying the cage and the bird has gone and to study the cage is not to study the bird – but still the body contains the divine in it.

The real way is to go within yourself and watch your own body from there - from The innermost of your being. There it is a tremendous joy – just to see it functioning, it's ticking. It's the greatest miracle that has happened in the Universe.

Why will the Human body age?
"Know yourself – that's the first duty of the human being to live a healthy life on this planet."
– M. Jayanth Reddy

Why all the planets including Earth, Sun and Sky and all heavenly bodies, galaxies are not wearing and tearing? Why the nature is never aging? Why only Human and living beings get older and die? What is the idea behind God's selfishness? I wonder only living creatures including us are all aging in this earth.

As new season starts, old leaves fall and new will arise along with frets accordingly. Further the cold season, Rainy season and summer season it will wear and tear. It will change with changeless state but no aging. Even with Humans also, there will be wear and tear. For example, inner body cells living on our intestines being renewed in every four to five days and red blood cells being replaced on average of 120 days. The skin is renewed in every 30 days and further the skeleton is renewed in every 90 days. And all proteins in the inside of the body including all organs clearing within 150 days. In total approximately 97 to 98% of the human body is renewed in 365 days and remaining 2% to 3% will get renew in due time. The same will happen with Nature too.

We humans are searching like blind people where the world is and what's our purpose in this world, where we stand and what we are. There are tens and thousands of researches in this world who couldn't help. New theories and discoveries of information about how aging occurs, what needs to be done to avoid aging. God made every life being as eternal. There is no birth and death. It's the atman only. Physical body changes. Man dies – means physical body dies. But Atma remains. This is biggest growing unanswered question by our modern people. Now we will discuss in more detail about how to prevent life. We forgot the wisdom of our past great grandfathers, great fathers' lineage and died old fashioned.

I understand that the God's wish is that we must labor, the physical body movement cultivates and survival physical work. But today, we are not doing any workout, physical exercise. Without wear and tear of the body parts and the movement of body parts, we will end up deteriorating our health. Its nature. Sun goes from east to west with earth circularly rounding it. For instance, if earth stops movement, or air stops flowing – the consequence are very many and disastrous too. I hope everyone will understand by this comparison. The same with human body as well. We must move muscles, ligaments, joints and inner organs – for smooth and synchronous functioning of the human body. Otherwise, the body will invite serious diseases and loose its charm and become diseased.

There are always two equal and opposite forces working in synergy on the universe. Like Father and mother, cold and hot. Weather is having a synchronized cycle called seasons. God has given us right food to eat and digest to be healthy -like intake of fruits, vegetables, herbs etc. There are antioxidant foods with which help to eliminate many diseases. Modern society mainly ignored the God given gift of natural food. In ancient times, monks and sages are very much qualified in solving many health-related problems and curing diseases with food. Ancient medical trees, herbs, fruits, vegetables and the knowledge of this is destroyed by the religion and the selfish ends of the rulers. A few God's given gifts are still left in the world and it's my primary responsibility to share that with you all.

According to me, no one have compared humans and planets and further I can simply believe that not a single person in this universe is following and maintaining one's own health – mainly because of our own modern societal rules, which made our life's venerable and miserable.

One must know oneself first. You know yourself – that's the first duty of the human being to live a healthy life on this planet.

In the astrology and astronomy effects on human being chapter, I discussed in detail with Mr. P.V.R. Rayudu (Ex-Senor Scientist, DRDL) about the effect of nature and its influence on human body. How the astronomy and astrology play a role in the well-being of the human being is discussed at length there. Mr. Rayudu authored several books on this subject and is a well-known name in this subject.

Astronomy and Astrology – Its effects on human Life

Astronomy and Astrology and Human life.

The Universe contains an infinite number of Solar systems, many of them are very much greater than our own. As we realize this, our vision will widen, our minds expand, and our hearts become filled with wonder and reverence for that Great Supreme and Unknowable Power that is the primary cause of all the glory that fills spare. But no amount of speculation concerning other solar systems can reveal the true state of things in the broad expanse of the heavens. It therefore become more profitable to us at our present stage to confine our attention to the Solar System of which we form a part, leaving the fixed start with their immense distances and magnitude out of our consideration. If we expand our imagination and think of our Sun as being in the center of an enormous circle, extending millions of miles into space and embracing the whole System, we might begin to realize what the conference of a Solar System means. It will be well to ponder over this wonderful system. The whole Solar System was a vast heated nebulous mass which cooling down, threw away huge portions which finally became planets or worlds, forming a complete planetary system resolving round the Sun.

Astronomy gives a knowledge of the celestial bodies, their magnitudes, motions, distances, periods, sizes, weight, order etc.

Astrology is a unique method of interpretation of the correlation of planetary influence. This implies that there is a constantly moving relationship between the very large moving objects of the universe such as the Sun, Moon and planets and the small moving objects such as human beings and animals.

The question of the scientific origin of Astrological knowledge has been the subject of controversy. Modern scientists have not hesitated to brand astrology as a superstition, and even its kindest critics refer to it as pseudo-science.

A knowledge of facts, laws and proximate causes, gained and verified by exact observation and correct thinking also, the Sum of Universal knowledge - an exact and systematic statement or classification of knowledge concerning some subjects or group of subjects, or any department of knowledge in which the results of investigation have been systematized.

If this be a correct definition of Science, then indeed is Astrology the greatest of all Sciences, Science its percepts and its formula were accumulated and established over a period of thousands or years of observation by man. Astrology is the oldest of all sciences. It is the real Science of the Starts. It is a Science of all Science, the key to all knowledge. It is indeed a synthesis of all branches of knowledge. It includes in its various ramifications such modern sciences as Astronomy, Medicine, Biology, Chemistry, Physics, and Psychology and many others.

The first principle upon which the Science of Astrology rests is, that the whole universe is what the term implies - a unity and that a law which is found manifestation in one portion of the universe must also be equally operative throughout the whole. The consequent to this major premise is that our own Solar System being a complete whole, those laws which are operative among the major constituents of that system, viz... The planetary bodies are also in force among the lesser components of the same system – to which us, and the other objects on this earth, whether solid, fluid or gaseous whether human, animal, vegetable or mineral.

The Second principle is, that by a study of the motions and relative positions of the planets the operations of these laws may be observed, measured and determined from these two first principles, aided by present day observation and a mind capable of metaphysical grasp of the metaphysical significance of phenomenal, the whole science of Astrology can be deduced. It is a mistaken for too prevalent when among thoughtful and unprejudiced people to suppose that, the present interest in Astrology is merely the decadent revival of so ancient superstition, based entirely on accepted tradition.

Nevertheless, since truth is the same in all the times, the learning of the ancients is of the greatest value to the modern students. Indeed. The astrologers who had to depend entirely on the first principles given above would certainly have a herculean task before him of observation, tabulation and induction before he would be even so well equipped and intelligently applies its principles.

The claims of Astrology are, that offers first and foremost a means of general character study entirely suppressing the combined advantages of ordinary anthropological methods, being at once more comprehensible and more subtle. Secondly. And this is pre— eminently its greatest, divine use, it's a means for the unbiased examinations of one's own character, and the most effective means of strengthening it. Thirdly, a knowledge of and seasons appropriate for certain works, and a means of testing one development of character. Lately and lastly though unfortunately by many made firstly and solely a means to some extent indeed, with those specially fitted, to a very remarkable extent - of forecasting future events.

It is true that Astrological science in all its implications extends into deep and far reaching metaphysical and philosophical domains, but after all what Science does not? The mathematical concepts of great Scientists like Einstein have already crossed the border from the domains of fixed form, and materialistic limitation into so—called fourth dimensional territories. Why should Scientists therefore, scoff at the implications contained in Astrology?

Astrology, while embracing all other Sciences was divided by the ancient Scientists into main sections

- That which dealt with the observation and recording of the relative position and motions of the celestial bodies in time.
- That which dealt with the observation and recording the correspondences between these positions and

   a) Natural phenomena occurring on the earth, such as weather, trees, earth quakes, floods and volcanic eruptions, growth and evolution of plant and animal life.

   b) Human physical phenomena such as Childbirth, death, menstruation of the female illness, disease, accident,

   c) Human psychological phenomena, as love, hate, envy, jealous, sex urge, avarice, greed and the physical actions resulting from these emotional states such as mating, murder, robbery, plunder, rape, combats and wars.

Of these two divisions of Astrological Scientific research that which dealt with the mere observance of the relative motions the celestial bodies (Astronomy) was considered as incidental. It was a first step toward the acquisition of the real knowledge - the only knowledge which really mattered, "the knowledge of the man, his origin and his destiny".

The First division - Astrology is today as a Science, because modern scientists with and of mechanical devices, continued and extended the observations of the ancient star scientists. The second division is not so recognized simply because on account of rank prejudice and skepticism, it has been ignored completely by present day Scientists who have made no attempt whatever to study and rationalize it. And yet there is no logical reason for this.

Certainly, there are few well known facts occurring in nature and falling within the scope of the second diversion of Astrological knowledge, which would seem to indicate that further investigation along this path would conform that other findings of the ancient scientists. Of these natural facts there are there which are outstanding

1. There does exist a correspondence because the phases of the Moon and the tides (Natural phenomena).
2. There does exist a correspondence between the phases of the Moon and the Menstrual periods of the female (Human Physical phenomena).
3. There does exist a correspondence between the periods of the Full Moon and the new Moon and the intensity of disturbance among the Insane (Human Psychological phenomena).

One of these facts happens to fall within the scope of each of the three subdivisions of the second section of Astrology indicated above. If these correspondences are true of the Moon is not rather presumptions to discord the rules set down by ancient Astrologers concerning the correspondences, which after many years of observation, they found to exist between the relative positions of the other planets and starts and the thoughts and actions of normal Men and Women? After all these observations and records were made by the same Astrologers, who first catalogued all the fixed starts. Who tabulated the distances and relative motions of the planets, their orbits and their periods of revolution, and who calculated with astonishing precision, the cycle of the equinoxes? Surely these men were intellectual giants, and their deductions at present merit investigation.

Astrology as a matter of fact, is the knowledge derived from the observation and study of the celestial bodies of which our earth is one in order to determine all possible relationships or correspondences which may exist between them and this search on which we have our being. Such observations surely should not confine to mere mathematical measurements calculations of time, space, volume and mass but should concern itself also will all other relationships which might concern ably exist. To simply dismiss as impossible any suggestion of correspondence between these time space measurements and the events which occur on this Earth or elsewhere is to willfully close the path to an interesting and scientific adventure.

Though the earnest knowledge of Astrology dates to mists of antiquity, lives and grows and needs constant representation in the light of current research. AS certain treatments have been believed to be most effective in field of Medical Science and later further experience changes these ideas and difference of opinion are then acknowledged, development of this Science requires or rather demands a full-scale research. One of the greatest handicaps of modern astrology is work has been done mainly by Isolated researchers, thus affording little opportunity for building this work into a solid body opinion.

Secondly many astrologers to carve a clear line through points of controversy indulge in oversimplification.

Thirdly the writers of paper astrology do not hesitant to bestow upon their remarks the technical name of Astrology. As such the depths of over supplication are now reached. Since the average educated period has never read a good book on astrology but has formed his opinion from its travesty thus found in print, the Science has been further discredited.

The entire basis of Astrology rests on the premise that the "Pattern" of a person correlation with the planetary pattern of his birth moment along with the rising Ascendant. The pattern at times, will, exterior, as "Events" the accuracy of these which can be in earlier life gives the astrologers the belief that tendencies deduced from calculation of future dates may be expected to evaluate as certain types of happenings in later life.

Whatever is born or done at a time has the qualities of that moment of time. In as much as a man identifies himself with the physical self and the physical world about him. so, he is in dissoluble part of it and subject to the changing pattern as formed by the planets in their orbits only by the recognition of that he senses as greater than himself can he himself to what beyond the terrestrial pattern. Constant motion of planets and that tremendous impact of their rays on the sensory nerves of the human body is responsible for the multifold changes in human behaviors, mental rake up, thought, conduct, health and everything that matters.

The Planets do influence man. When the earth is called into present shape by the Solar influences, where is the logic of suggesting that bodies on surface are not affected by them? A trifling change in weather through solar causes brings neuralgia, headache, bronchitis, sore eyes, and fever. Smallpox, cholera. Dysentery. Plague and a host of other disease too numerous to detail. War menace is a striking illustration of planetary influence. Our temper and moods depend upon the secretions of ductless glands. Fear is a matter or endocrine secretions. Indecision is a matter of thymus; genius is a matter OE thyroid Sun's cycles of behavior have their corresponding effects on those glands and their secretions and consequently on human.

Feel has a larger range than any of the other Faculties. Not only can objective things be sensed by touch. But we can also feel InviSible elements as heat, Cold and planetary vibrations. As planetary vibrations of varying character are continually exerting an influence which is taken up by our sensory news with the resulting bodily reactions, mental attitudes and moods. Therefore, it is possible that solar, lunar and stellar energies supply the cells through the media of the nerves their emotively. Different planetary vibrations, astrologically described as Yogas or aspects supply different sensory stimuli, accordingly the vibrations defer in wave lengths, Intensity, frequency etc.,

Radiations from starts and planets can affect the future destiny of an individual at conception. The great ancient Hindu astrologers propounded the importance of conception time much before the birth of the European civilization. Since conception time is difficult to be noted, the ancient Hindu "Maharishis" visualized, their divine insight and Intuition, that the sign at the actual birth time planetary configuration would be the Ascendant.

At the conception time and Moon would be in the sign of birth Ascendant and hence it was postulated that the horoscopes are the planetary configurations at birth time should be judged? From the Moon sign considering it as Ascendant in addition to the actual Birth time Ascendant.

The planets are merely reflectors or transmitters of light and solar energy. The Solar and planetary rays — radio like waves — affect biological and psychological processes. The rays of influence are unseen vibrations. They era not perceptible to the physical eyes. Human sight has its I Imitations. Therefore, the rays of influence can be cognized by other senses and means; for instance, the vibrations of Saturn are slow and hence things of corresponding nature are attributed to him and events during Saturn's periods do not occur fatly as compared to the events during the other first moving planets.

When the Sun and Moon are in conjunction, they are concentrating their Forces on the same part of globe at the same time and accounts for the abnormal conditions and does affect a Child born during conditions of this nature. For, witness our own bodies, we have innumerable glands whose work is the secretion of hormones. These are forever adjusting themselves in harmony with our chemically changing environment without, and are responsible for our emotions, desires, mental balance, rate of growth, and length of life on this planet. It but commonsense to say that the planetary positions of the Sun and the Moon which affect the sea water causing are bound to affect all the store of fluids on the surface of the earth or contained in vegetable kingdom or in human beings. The blood is not only a fluid but contains the same salts that are dissolved in the ocean and that too practically in the same proportion.

Hindu astrologers have given predictions for each day of the lunar month. For the eighth day, that is when the Sun and the Moon are 90 Degrees apart, they have said that this eight day removes the diseases or cures the ailments. On this day, Sun and the Moon, being 90 degrees apart, diminish each other's attractions on the fluids. The blood in the human beings remains thus comparatively undisturbed state from the outside influences and any medicine newly started on this day is bound to be more effective if at so properly and that is why there is the importance of this day.

From a gravitational and tactical point of view, the forces and magnitude of attraction between the earth and the planets in indeed tremendous. This must be continually varying due to the planets continually varying distances from the Sun and Moon and another constellation. The influence of planets upon mankind is undoubted. In a horoscope, the Sun the Moon and the Lagna or Ascendant represent the soul, the Mind and respectively of an individual. The Sun may be visualized as the dispenser of the various cosmic matter and the Moon as the mixer of this matter whole the Ascendant may be taken as a catalytic agent. The other planets are of course, symbols for interpreting these cosmic influences.

Astrologically when the Sun, the Moon and planets enter different constellations, their respective radiations vary and produce corresponding changes in the weather. Climate is regulated by the movements and Influences of the planets. Consequently, the influences of climate are clearly receptable. If there is any factor in the constitution of man and his temperaments which vitally influences him for work or for laziness, for strength or for ability, for intelligence or for dullness, is the climate. Those instances suggest that between the various atmospherically influences and the vital activity of the human nerves there seems to be a connection.

Measles, smallpox etc. are associated with the planet Mara. Whenever Mars makes his closest approach to the earth Martian epidemics should manifest. The menses of a woman sets in every month, when the Moon is in an *upacharya* (3rd, 6th, 10th, 11th houses) from the Ascendant that the menses are due to the interaction of Mars and the Moon. According to

Gochara or the Transit system, the noon passing through the different signs from his own projection in birth chart is said to make the native's psychological reactions differ on different days. On one day one is subject to serious facts of depress and on another day to strong sexual urges, on a third to creative thought and the next to fits of illness. Some lunatics or neurotic people on or some-tines even the normal rational people seem to have tides of irrationality rise and fall within them according to the waxing and waning of the Moon. All diseases and specially, Skin diseases. Insanity and epilepsy were believed to be subject to the Influence of the Moon, mental Planet. Diseases get more virulent in their efforts at the time of the New Moon. When the tidal forces are great at the time of the New Moon, they are enough to supply the spark to bring out conditions for an earthquake to happen or the gravitational pull of planets with that of the Sun and tends to create conditions for the occurrence of an earthquake. Moon has a definite effect on the periodically of Human births.

What we call "Raja Yogas" are certain special dispositions of planets affecting the combined radiation now of birth in such a way that the native would become great, famous and outstanding. For example, "Gaja Kesar Yoga" formed by the conjunction of square or Jupitar and Moon in a birth chart gives a beautiful life to the native provided they are not afflicted on Ill placed or weak in the horoscope with respect to the ascendant.

It is a remarkable thing that the important events during the entire life happen at astrologically important movements when the "DASAS AND BHUKTAS" (astrological time measure) as per Hindu Astrology of powerful or weak planets operate. The dominant combinations in Hitler's horoscope is the disposition of Saturn in the 20th House and Mars in the 7th House, each expecting the other powerfully and Jupiter's befit however consigned to a minor position. Astrological textbooks say that and Saturn combination (which includes aspects also) in certain houses, subject of course, to the general strength or otherwise of the horoscope, is said to make the subject extremely aggressive. Mars in the house of death signifies violent end. Venus is supposed to rule marriage and the sex element and his presence in the 10th house executes passions and the person will be highly sexed. Mars in combination with Venus indicates more than one marriage, want of happiness from marriage etc. The association of Venus with Saturn, mars and Rahu (Dragon's Head) is always indicative of either want of happiness in domestic or over sexuality making one seek Illegal sex gratification.

Twins are alike sometimes and different sometimes, sometimes twins will have commons character and others different. Such as variations as a rule are due to slight difference in the time of birth. The word twin implies two entities coming into manifestations under the same planetary pattern. This also be extended to include two born approximately not exactly) for the same time regardless of parentage or environmental conditions of birth. In fact, the Important experience of two or three persons born on the name day but at different times and every in a different country likely to have a parallel significance, though one is a doctor, the other a banker and the third our Astrologer and at times the striking similarities may go to the extent that they look alike, both play the piano, have same name, both are accomplished swimmers, both have a chronic catarrhal condition of the threat, both have exceptional eyesight, the fathers of both are contractors and grandfathers of both have accidents to their feet followed by Infection and death, the father's mother due when the father is about 5 years old, both have two sisters and one brother and both are Interested In scientific study of astrology etc.

The ancient genius Hindu astrologers through their Divine insight and insight developed deep into that Astronomical phenomena with respect to the minute concept of time and laid down Astrological rules for different events in.

The life of human being and other species. They visualized the general events in human for every 24 seconds of difference in birth time and events with respect to the particular configuration of planets and ascendant at the time of birth. They have written down these events in advance on palm leaves in the so called Nadi Astrology in India, some of which are still prevalent in India. If the past events of a nature with respect to the parentage, coborns, partners, profession etc., can be judiciously searched and matched with those available on the palm leaves, the future events already written on the palm leaves for the particular nature would mostly and astoundingly come out there. Each Sign or Rasi is divided into 300 parts so that each part comes under the name of a "Nadi Amsa measuring 12 minutes of are in the sign or 43 seconds in time. This minute division the seed of destiny of an individual. If the correct Nadi is established, then there is a bird's eye view of the entire past including the past life and future of future of the person concerned. Each "Nadi Amsa" is further divided into two parts each of 6 minutes of arc in the sign or 24 seconds in time and general pattern of life is given. There are hundreds of Nadi Granthas as they're called in south India and "Samhitas" as they are called in North India and majority of them are not genuine ones. Nadis that are not based on astrological consideration but dole out predictions purporting to be astrological should be ignored by all well—wishers of astrology. It goes to the credit of "Satya Charya" a genuine Hindu Astrologer for this great discovery of Nadi system.

Nadi Amsa: Pressing at Navel point is India's traditional curing in ancient times. Indian monks used to press on Nadi Amsa i.e., on Navel - where there is to cure many diseases depending on timing of the day.

Each Nadi Amsa has got its own peculiar characteristic but can clearly indicate one's pattern of destiny. In relation to planetary positions, birth star etc. can give an idea of one's parentage, number of brother's sisters etc. A Nadi Amsa in an Ascendant within 6 minutes of relate to a birth star and certain other planetary situations can enable to predict future events with considerable accuracy. No astrologer of the present times has come forward to explain what the basis of Nadi Astrology is and how it is patterned.

In a very general sense without knowing the actual ascendant and planetary configuration, one is born during 0 degrees to 12' in a movable sign ascendant (in Aries cancer, Libra, Capricorn) or 29048' to 300 in a fixed sign ascendant (etc. Taurus, Leo, Scorpio, Aquarius) or 150 to 15212' in dial sign ascendant i.e. (Gemini, Virgo Sagittarius, Pisces), he will be born in a place near a river or sea in a rich family a worshipper of God, four good complexion, slightly corpulent; father famous and well placed in life and has two wives; native eldest son of the Second wife; brothers will be short lied' parents are early in life; helped by an uncle; get good and pleasing manners both grandfather and father highly fortunate; prosperity through lands; regards for God; three marriages;

First marriage 21st year; passionate; befriends higher ups in Government; of mild nature and good qualities'; protects a number of people; becomes very rich; first wife dies after giving birth to a Child; befriends higher ups in Government' of mild nature and good qualities' protects a number of people; becomes very first wife dues after giving birth to a Childs enters Government service in 21st year' 2nd marriage in 36th years and goes on loss of service in 30th year; 3rd marriage after 40th year; all issues born to the 3rd wife due two sons and one daughter have long general fortunate from birth to death. "Satya Charya" another of Nadi pattern of Astrology confirms that no astrological predictors should be given without knowing and the exact Amsa in the Ascendant. that is, without finding the exact degree and minute of the Ascendant for birth time up to 6 minutes off arc generally corresponding and matching to the past events of the nature and then only to proceed further to delineate the horoscope for future events with respect to the exact planetary configuration of the horoscope. Therefore, is evident that no horoscope should be read for the future events without knowing the past events and the background of the native. The future events should be given as per the social, economic, circumstantial, environmental background of the native.

Under the present times when the birth rate so fast, for example one birth almost every second In India one birth for almost every 3 Seconds In the world. It would be a herculean task for any present-day astrologer to judiciously predict any particular events and only general guidance can be given. Moon moves every 21/2 days through one sign and 12 positions would come for every month. Ascendant changes every two hours in a day. Sun, Venue, Mercury transits through each sign for 11/2 months. Jupiter remains in each sign for one year. The Nodes Rahu (Dragon's head) and Ketu (Dragon's head) cover each sign for every 11/2 years. Saturn is the slow-moving planet revolving in each sign once in 21/2 years. The others Uranus, Neptune considered by western Astrologers would be still slower in their motion. In a particular Year, particular month, particular day and with a particular Ascendant there would be 300 patterns of horoscopes are to be dealt with the same planetary configuration when the Ascendant is divided into 300 Amass i.e. when every 6 minutes of arcs of the complete 300 of the particular ascendant is considered and for all the 12 Ascendants in that particular day 3600 life patterns are to be analyzed. In particular year considering the movements of Moon & Sun and Ascendants Nadi Amsa of 6 minutes of arc, there would be 518400 different planetary and Ascendant configurations are to be studied. Hence it would be herculean task to delineate the life pattern of an individual precisely.

It was visualized by the ancient Hindu astrological sages that a particular region under the same latitude and longitude in each Nadi Amsa, the order of births would be 1 Deva Godly 2 Asura (Demonly) 24 humans, 10 beasts, 11 birds, 12 reptiles, 25 water beings 20 plants, 25 minerals totaling to 120 births. That is in a particular region general there would be 24 human births for every 4 a second's intervals. Assuming theoretically two males are born at the game day, month and year in India and America, the two males when they attain youth cannot go ahead with their amorous activities, with any girl in a similar fashion, due to the social and environmental conditions of the country. The Indian youth will be restricted in his love affairs and the American would go ahead with his sex activities with his beloved girl. Similarly, the life pattern of a particular region or country also would play a part while tallying results of persons in those areas. It would be a future exercise for an astrologer for an astrologer to have predicted a very affluent for a person in Japan before the atomic bomb explosion during the Second World War. Also, the predictions should not be the same for a person dwelling in a hut and a building though the two might have born nearly at the same time, day, month and year having same planetary configurations. The hut dweller might possess a motorcycle at the time when the other person in the building with a better rich background might buy a motor car. However, in both cases the life pattern and progress would be similar, and the astrologer should tell the results judiciously and intelligently.

At this junction, obviously the theories of 'Karma' and 'fate' come to play whatever man soweth, he reaps. The actions taken by pest life or in the previous birth would come forward giving the future results. Fates also are four types. Alterable good fate, alterable fate, unalterable good fate and unalterable bad fate. The scope for altering the alterable bad fate would also be built in.

In the planetary configuration for him if it meant for him and he would be ad versed and grinded by intelligent astrologer or any other person when the time comes. In case of unalterable bad fate, nothing could be done, and the fate takes own course even if one takes necessary earlier precautionary measures. In case of a motorcycle accident, the person having an alterable bad fate could come out with minor injury when advised in advance and taken necessary earlier precaution. In case of the person with an unalterable bad fate hardly listen to the advice and meet with a fatal injury. Even the fate also occurs with respect to the first person or second person or third person. In the motor cycle accident, the person himself may hit something and meet with the accident or another person coming in another motorcar may hit the person or neither of the two persons are involved and a third type of activity such as group clashes, earthquake etc. affect the person in accident.

It should be borne in mind then events happen only when the right time comes depending on the background. Here the three 'S' analogy of seed, soil and season can be understood profitably. The seed pattern will be same but when the correct soil and season come into operation only the seed grow and bloom into a tree. Similarly, the human seed would be the same depending on one's genes and past Live deeds and one's life pattern will grow accordingly when required circumstance come into play at the required times. Even enlightened 'Gurus' cannot save the person from bad fate, at best they can do probably to take on them the bad fate of their disciples and suffer themselves saving their disciples

But the 'Karma' to be performed in any case by somebody. It is told that when Jupiter is connected with the Ascendant, 5th house and 9th house. God's Grace would be there and most of the evils be averted, but however, this type of planetary configuration also would come when one is born depending on his actions, but his actions have no control over their results.

The ancient astrologers have attributed different significances to various planets and houses in a horoscope. For example, Venus is given signification of 'Arts ' and 12th house represents 'fret ' being the last house Ascendant. While giving 'Sthula' (Apparent), 'Sookshma' (intricate) and the 'Kaarana' (cause) aspects in the horoscope are to be seen. For example, 'Karana' planet for fine arts to Venus, the Lord the 12 houses would be 'Sookshma. And the planets in the house would appear only as 'Sthula 'in giving results say dancing. If Venus is totally afflicted in the horoscope, though the other two of the 12th lord and 12 house planets would not be able to give good results for Achieving in dancing. For example, even if the feet are fitted the person can dance provided the 'Karana' planet. Venus is strong and benefit without any affections. The Analogy of Electric Transformer in a housing Colony Electric meter in the house and electric bulb in the room can be compared to the 'Karana', 'Sookshma' and 'Sthula' respectively. If all the three are good, the light will come but if the electrical transformer has been spoiled the whole source is lost.

The day is past for writing a difference of Astrology, and no amount of argument will ever convince the sceptic who either too indolent or too perverse to investigate a science which claims to explain law that govern all thing. The best test that can be applied, to as to all other subjects where first—hand knowledge is required, is that of experience. Reason thought and experience basis from which the system adopted to give Astrological predictions is to be built- However many still consult astrology for genuine guidance or due to curiosity to know what in store for them in future.

Summing up, Astrology is not only a most forecasting intellectual study but a remarkable tool for sculpturing the Soul, Body and Mind and the fringe of the future events. Astrology cannot be called a science in narrow science because science deals with material objects. Yet Astrology is based on scientific data. Astrology is an applied Science and therefore become an art also. The only thing is, one should not attempt to make astrology fatalistic and use as a mean in evading the responsibilities of free will, science. Most of the present astrologers have not got the ability and institution to develop deep into the most intricacies of the planetary influences their positioning and the birth chart and subsequent motions in the cycle persons and to rectify the birth time to the correct correspondence to match with the past like events with respect to background of the native. However, it is a fact established from times immemorial that Astrology is a science and the Art in the hand of an honest sincere, intelligent and intensively astrologers to predict the future events converting the effects of the planets, houses on ascendant and the configuration at birth with subsequent planetary motions through the emotional physiological, social economical circumstantial. Egoistical environmental, psychological conditions. Thus, Astrology definitely guide the realms of human life.

Chi Power or Prana

Healthy human being is primarily or fundamentally based on life energy. Life energy is equivalent term being described in Sanskrit as "Prana". When this life energy is less or not adequate, the function of all the connectors of organs/circulation/nervous system (psycho/physic) is lesser. Consequently, innumerable diseases out of modern lifestyle attack the human system and the mankind is on the verge of being victimized and has become vulnerable to the various diseases.

When our life is powered by artificial ideas instead of the true feelings of our life energy, it draws, consumes, exhausts and causes damage to our life energy which leads to Chi's steady decline of our body, mind and spirit. Weak life energy means a weak physical and mental condition that prevents us from living a normal healthy and peaceful life. People who want to live a real and better life must first learn how to rebuild and restore their life energy by Chi exercises.

Chi exercises are said to be saviors of restoring and improving the psychological and physical health and longevity of the present-day people. Though there are number of alternative methods which lure people with immediate cure or permanent cure of diseases, people have been becoming victims of the side effects and other consequences during the medication.

Any method must recognize the defunct system of the patient before treating the patient. Here with Chi exercises/life energy exercises, we could reach at the deceased defunct system of the human body and starts curing it from the elementary or root stage. Of course, it depends on everyone's system of body; hence the Chi exercises may differ from one individual to another individual.

Undoubtedly, Chi is going to play a bigger role in the world of health and longevity. Even in Chi, cosmos or like Mother Nature or the weather/sunny /blue sky days and unpredictable stormy events co exists in our life. as it is ingrained, everything in the cosmos is interrelated and interconnected.

Chi is constantly turning, changing and reacting just like the force that governs the weather. Change is a natural part of life energy sustaining itself. The question is whether the change in your life serve to help balance and sustain your equilibrium or whether the changes cause disharmony and distress. The condition of your Chi determines and provides the answer.

We are all made up of Chi, because our Chi follows in the same way the entire universe moves. Hence, we are an integral part of the universe. For that matter, we are all born into cosmos and interconnected with life energy.

Chi: Chi means energy, which is generated from the 11/2 inches below the navel point. In China, people call Chi as energy which deliver from below the navel. There are several exercises to condition Chi Energy, whose Point which is 11/2 inches below navel.

The following are some of the breathing exercises that helps us to know your Chi.

Breathing exercises have been practiced in several countries in their ways. For instance, in Indian context we call breathing exercise as Pranayama. Chinese say Chi, Japanese utter it as Qi and Koreans say Ki etc.,

Since ages, dating back to 4th Century B.C, people have been practicing breathing exercises all over the world in different ways.

Today, there is an innovative progress in the study of breathing exercises, especially, there are 16 departments including institute of atomic energy of the Chinese academy of natural science, experimented with the physical and physiological effects of breathing exercises on different individuals for 100 to 1000 times; they are able to prove that breathing helped them tremendously physically and mentally than non-breathing exercises.

Since seventies, a few foreign research units, departments carried out research on breathing exercises, body channels, meridian of human body and the nature of Prana, Chi, Qi, Ki in a multidisciplinary and comprehensive method.
I have read a discussion made in international symposium of breathing exercise held in Prague, Morocco and Toronto (Canada) in the year 1973.

In 1975, the Marsh European University in Switzerland made a comprehensive study of breathing exercises from a physiological, biochemical and psychologic standpoint. About 3000 students have graduated from that university and published many research papers in 1976 in journal of biofeedback magazine from USA and did a special study on Qi, Chi, Ki, etc.,

With the increasing research information, many research departments were established in Europe, Asia, north and South America.

Medical research on a few diseases I would like to mention....

1. Nervous system
2. Cardiovascular system
3. Digestive system
4. Endocrine system
5. Respiratory system

How nervous system is being helped by breathing exercises.

My experience and study have proved that quietness eliminates tension in the cerebral cortex, reinforces its adjusting capacity and improves the function of all human organs. Comprehensive study by many scientists found that the electroencephalographic (EEG) waves from various parts of cortex were different in their volts, after breathing exercise the voltage increases as much as 150 to 180 micro volts with synchronous increases in electroencephalogram (ECG) voltage in all areas of the cortex. This shows that breathing exercise will bring the electric activity of nerve cells to a high degree of orderliness. Experiments also revealed that after exercises, patients with high blood pressure showed a relative weakening of reaction in the sympathetic nerve, while that of the parasympathetic nerve was strengthened and the activity of dopa-S-hydroxyls was lowered, another sign of the weakening excitation in the sympathetic nerve.

How cardiovascular system is being helped by breathing exercises. Breathing exercises promote blood circulation by dilating the capillaries and strengthen the pulse. The patient's heartbeat slows down after breathing exercises; with an increase in cardiovascular output when inhaling deeply and increases in returning blood volume during the deep exhaling. The burden of the heart can be lightened. Though breathing exercises, sufferers of hypertension and arteriosclerosis will suffer no further hypertrophy or enlargement of their hearts and recovery from arrhythmia.

The way digestive system and its function are improved through breathing exercise.

During abdominal breathing in Chi or Pranayama, breath control or breath holding method, organs in the abdominal cavity seems to be massaged rhythmically. The diaphragm's range of movement is three or four times more than during regular breathing. The rhythmic change of the infra-abdominal pressure massages the Stomach, Intestine, Liver, Gallbladder, and Pancreas, thereby causing an increase of gastrointestinal peristalsis and thus of juice secretion and a decrease of abdominal blood stagnation. Improves digestion and absorption functions. Breathing exercises promotes good appetite and helps complete assimilation.

There are all a few points and techniques I have mentioned about the effects on diseases, but there are 100s of benefits regarding curing diseases. This book will address and give adequate information about breathing exercises in a very precise manner.

The method of breathing exercises:

a. One must adjust the body according to the posture.
b. Second is preparing the mind or keeping the mind concentrated on the breath

c. Third one is adjusting the breath itself, especially on the process of inhalation and exhalation.

According to the methods and techniques of Chi, QI, Ki or Pranayama – Breathing exercises have proved to definite and positive effect on each organ and all systems of the body and mind. Further cures all diseases and maintains good health and well-being. Breathing exercises.
Breathing exercises in sitting.
Simple Pranayama.
Close your right nose with right thumb and leave all the air from left   nostril and then breath in through left nostril and close the left nostril and leave all the air from right nostril and close the right nostril. Continue for 10 minutes daily after bowel movement.

During this breathing in and out pattern, all your mind's concentration should be on your breath only. Note: This breathing exercise should be done with eyes closed. Further, your breath in and breath out should not exceed 6 respirations a minute.

Breathing exercise in walking

Breathe in (control air) for 10 steps and breath out, control air and walk 10 steps.

Breathe in while walk 5 to 10 steps, and breath out while walking next 10 steps.

Breath in (control air), punches at solar level for 10 to 20 times and relax for 10 seconds and breath out while punching 10 to 20 times. This exercise can be done in standing or horse stance.

Breathing exercise in standing position

Stand straight and keep palm on the navel (men to use Left palm and women to use right palm). And keep the right hand on the left hand. Bend your body 45 degrees forward, press your navel area with palm for 10 to 15 times while breathing in, and breathe out while coming back to straight position. Feel that perineum is relaxing. One should do these 10 times every day.

Stand and keep left hand on navel and keep right hand over the left hand. Press hard while breathing in and breathe out and relax. One should do these 36 times a day.

Breathing Exercises sitting on chair

One

Sit on a chair comfortably, relax and close your eyes. After half a minute, breath in and feel, believe that toes of your left leg are relaxing, then right toe – feel and believe that they are relaxing. Slowly move your observation to upwards, feel that your left foot is relaxing, and then right foot is relaxing. Then left ankle and right ankle; then left calf and right calf, then left Chin and right Chin. Feel relaxed and believe with breathing. Slowly move further upwards, feel that your left knee is relaxing and then the right knee, and then left thigh and right thigh, then lower back, lower abdomen ; then upper back and then chest then left shoulder and then right shoulder; then left triceps and then left triceps, then right biceps right elbow and left biceps left elbow, left forearm and then right forearm, left wrist and right wrist, then left four fingers and then right four fingers, then left thumb and right thumb and feel that whole body is relaxing. With each breath you must experience that the whole body is relaxing. Wake up after 2 minutes of blocking your thoughts.

Two

Sit with legs crossed and keep tow hands (palms) stick together and breath in with nose (tongue stick to the top of the mouth) and breath out with mouth.

Please note that while breathing in you must keep tongue touching the roof of your mouth. These breathing exercises should be done with eyes open.

Breathing exercises lying down

Lie down in Shavasana(Corpse Pose) with hands besides thighs and palms facing sky.

1. Breath in and breath out and feel your two legs are relaxing
2. Breath in and breath out and feel your two hands are relaxing
3. Breath in and breath and feel your whole body is relaxing. One should do above mentioned three breaths 10 sets every day.

Lie down like above Shavasana keep 5 to 10 kg weight sand bag/rice bag on lower an abdomen.

Breath in – raise your abdomen slowly, up to the maximum and breath out while bringing down the abdomen. One should do this for 10 minutes daily.

Asana: Asana means posture. Indian people practice Yoga and each posture is called an Asana. These Yoga Asana are therapeutic postures people will do and stay on each and every position for 10 seconds to 1 minute depending on these disease and pain.

Shavasan (Corpse Pose): Shavasana is the posture of relaxation. Shava means dead body and Asana means posture. In this Asana, one will lie down flat on the floor and palms facing the sky.

Every human being is born to live long life i.e., 200 years to 800 years, actual age of human is 1000 years. God made us after many generations of animal's diversification to human life. Today's modern life is not even living 10% of that life. I came out with very in-depth and profound study of life of human being to enlighten how one can live life in this present world. I have read many books about long life of human being and known through great priest/masters of martial arts and known through people who lived 100 + years, that human can live at least 200 years without any problem and even with present modern life. In one of the oldest books I read, during 700B.C. one Mr. Patriarch Peng is mythical being and he has attained a fabulous longevity of 767 years of age when Shang dynasty nearing ending i.e., 1123 B.C. and recently in the year 1677 Mr. lee Chen born and died in the year 1933 he has attained 256 years, Chikung master from China lived 202 years, his first photograph was taken on his 200 th birthday in Shanghai and is kept in museum. And so, I want everyone to know to learn the system of living long life.

So presently the whole world is limiting the life of human being and transferring the life into materialistic world (modern world) without aiming for protecting the life - in which only one can live only one life. By spoiling the body many people are prone to achieve a rich man status, honor, saving properties which doesn't help to long life/ healthy life. Millions of people have done same way and the process of accumulating the wealth and running behind materialistic success - goes on destroying the body for generations. You can notice that many scientists, business magnets and many renowned people from all walks of life died at early age. To cite few examples,

Vivekananda born on 1863 and died on 1902 (39years).

Albert Einstein born on 14th March 1879 and died on 18th April, 955 (76years).

Isaac Newton born on 4th Jan 1643 and died 1727.

William Shakespeare born on 23rd April. 1564 and died 23rd April, 1616 (80years).

Abraham Lincoln born on Feb 12th of 1809 and died on 1865 (56 years)

Walt Disney born during 1906 and died 1966 (60 years)

Karl F. Benz Born on 1844 and died 1929 (85years).

JRD Tata born on 1904 and died on 1992 (88 years).

Dhirubai Ambani Born on 1932 and died on 2002 (70 years)

These above said people were on mission to achieve desired heights in various fields but poor concentration on health. They treated their body/life as salved of their human body.

With the above examples we can understand that past and present people and their lifestyle. Its every Human being's responsibility to understand Human body. The human body is a miniature universe in itself, and one has to exercise regularly to regulate all 5 organs with co-ordination of flow of blood to every part of anatomy and nerve system.

Human beings cannot sustain high quality of life and live long only by food alone. He/she must understand human body and its functions fully. Millions of people died in the past, though they are high scholars, Nobel Prize winners, Top doctors, scientists - we lost world famous people. They couldn't understand well about this Body and human system.

Every person has a potential for perfect health. It may require little effort and dedication towards exercise, but the rewards are often tremendous.

It is the time for the people of the world to realize a look for regular exercises to promote better health and longevity. It is not the theory that make them the world healthy nor the knowledge that make them healthier nor the money - but it must be the practical implementation.

Even in the past all high status, high honored scholarly people of the world passed away even though they are high skilled in the academically.

I have come out with many ancients' secret exercises (breathing, organ cleaning, medicinal exercise, physical exercises with yin and yang effective acupressure, meridian points and organ impulses. To help the world to attain fabulous age with peaceful/cheerful life, I am sharing this information that have learned by begging, borrowing and stealing from various countries grandmasters/healers of the world after their personal achievement from their ancestors.

Human being can live without food for month or so without water a week or so but without air/breath 2 or 30 minutes. With control of breath we regulate the organs to function systematically in specific pattern – and this is the secret to attain long life. It is like a control of seconds, and obviously hours, days, weeks, months, years will control of itself.

 The secret is the breathing from the abdomen to the point below the 1.1/2 inch to 2 inches below the navel. Indians says Prana, Chinese says Chi, Japanese and Koreans says Ki. In many other countries says thee, Chi, Kee, dim Mak, Meing Mein, Tan Teing, and (Indian says) Kundalini and all are the same. The Taoists believe that the original source of being and life is situated and comes from the point in the abdomen called Tan Tein, the medical science believe that it is profound in the lumber vertebra at the point opposite to the kidneys.

This breathing (Chi/Prana/Ki) exercises were developed way back – almost more than 6000 years ago, and they are based on original human being and nature's rules with the ultimate aim of preventing and healing disease and healthy life – thereby achieve longevity. This knowledge was handed over to the people from generations to generations through grandmasters priests and masters including Buddha, Taoists masters from father to son and master to disciple since then this knowledge was passed on to the world one by one country.

During that period about 5000 to 6000years back priest and masters used to clean dirt from the bones, tendency, muscles, and organs and get new hair and new skin. In ancient days healers/priests and masters/yogis treated illness no matter how many kinds of diseases one may have all will vanish. Hence life consequently prolonged through balancing of yin and yang (+ve and -ve energies). In the year 500 B.C Many of the masters and priests used to have super natural powers and can levitate the body in air and were walking on trees/water and travel more than 1000 to 2000rniles a day, send messages to people 1000's of miles through their minds and healed any type of disease. This can be possible even today by rediscovering the lost ancient knowledge. Many scholars, doctors, scientists in the present world may say that these are unscientific and unproven, but you trust me that those who say are the people who never understood the pre-history and the power of our ancestors. Even Chi/Ki power is also unproven, and people consider it unscientific, but many masters move the objects without touching them. Also, they demonstrated the ability to hit the physical body form a very far distance. I have seen this in Asia and Europe during my visits there. Further I also heard that Taoist masters create rain and even stop rain by their power.

Life and Death of Human being

First The fact that whatsoever is born in this world in this stream of time will certainly die. In the realm of time, death is a phenomenon that is definite, certain. In this realm of time, death is unavoidable. Whatsoever is born in the realm of time is bound to perish.

The truth is that creation and destruction are opposite poles of the same phenomenon. The moment something is created, it has already begun to perish. The moment someone is born, his journey towards death has already began. Mahavira once said, "man's life is like dew drop balanced on the tip of a blade of grass, whether it falls now or in a short time from now, it will certainly fall. It must fall. Further many also said life is like mere bubble, it blasts now or later.

Millions of people in this world throughout their life, live less and spend more time and energy safeguarding against death, they run, they scramble, they earn money, they acquire fame, they build houses with high and strong walls, with big safes, they make all sorts of arrangements for their security for one reason only they don't want to die.

But eventually they do die. All their safety measures fail, all their precautions prove to be futile. All their efforts, all their endeavors, all their attempts prove to be vain.

Billions of people have just wasted their lives in their way of fighting against death. The most important aspect of everyone in this world is to be fit, regularly take time to repair, thereby staying healthy physically and mentally.

Millions of people are worried about external life but not about internal life i.e., their inner fitness, inner organs' fitness, inner neurological fitness, inner wellbeing. This will only happen when everyone put in regular exercise in every level from cell to organ and to the muscles. Only then one can delay death and longevity will perish. Many people think external life, like the wealth, money and they put entire life in accumulating money as if it is secure and permanent with which they can fight against the momentariness of things and this is one of the humans' basic disease.

Take the example of Andrew Carnegie. He left billions of dollars behind and till the end of his life he was discussing business on the phone when he breathed his last. A biographer of Andrew Carnegie wrote I haven't seen even a single moment in Carnegie's life when I could say that he was really living. Every moment he was only earning. Perhaps he was the richest man on earth, but in a sense, nobody was poorer than he was. Because he did not know the thrill of life, he couldn't be touched by any waves of life. Often his friends would say to him, "what are you going to do with all the money that you are accumulating? "and he would say, "wait, once I am finished with making money, I will start living. "But the earning never finished, and the living never began.

This is addiction of life earning money. You might have seen people in money gambling in Casino.

How they spend money in losing and earning is their joy of life. It is same as earning even you may be the richest man in the world. Don't make mistakes, take time for life. Be healthy. Take time for repairing the life.

Do anyone in the world monitor or notice regularly of his/her organs and their deficiencies/weaknesses day by day. Do anyone notice their body is weakening day by day. Their ligaments, limbs, muscles are unknowingly getting weakened by not exercising and strengthening

If this physical body, inner and outer, is not monitored and not controlled by you, it will be by itself and will attract many diseases. Fighting with yourself in strengthening is only the best way of exploring the best life and it is the most fundamental challenge you need to think.

If you don't control your body, body will control you and same as if you don't digest the food the food will digest you.

Human Body and the Universe

"God is in sweat. The more you sweat, the nearer you will be to God". M. Jayanth Reddy

Ying and Yang – Relationship of Human body and the Universe

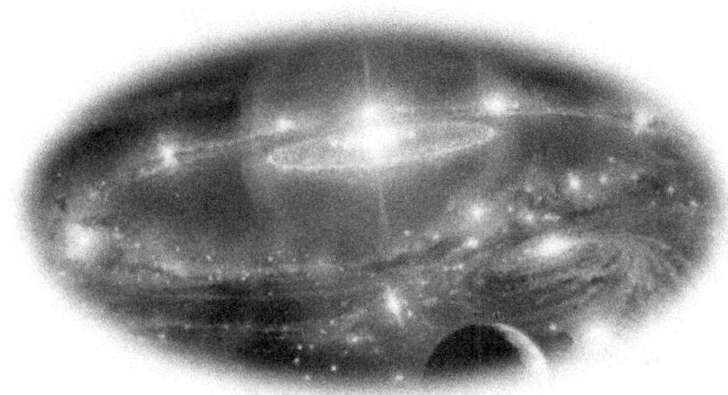

The human-life runs primarily on with two organic principles which spread all parts of the body called Yin and Yang, the union of which the human being is made, and life depends. The Yin and Yang are quite opposite polarities and keenly reflected in our daily life, e.g., the union of man and woman and merging of day into night.

In China, people call the Yin and Yang, in India the term we associate with is Hatha (Hatha Yoga). In India it was thought that God and the Devil have equal abilities and coexisted in the universe like opposite forces - South Pole and North Pole of a magnet.

The Yin and Yang was first noticed during 3rd and 4th century BC that this universe is serving through balance, if there is any imbalance in nature then automatically results in earthquake, tsunami, cyclone etc., will be produced.

The Yin and Yang balance is required for good health. Yang foods will increase the body temperature and yin foods will lower the body temperature. Yin and Yang exist in interdependence, and Yin and Yang balance and control each other, these Yin and Yang relationship is between five element and astrology of time. In ancient India and China, many healers, Taoists, Yogis and Priests treated illnesses - no matter how many kinds of diseases one may have all will vanish, and hence life consequently prolonged.

The Five Elements

The theory of the five elements was originally espoused in the Neijing (Nei China) the yellow emperor during 3rd B.C. and was intended to represent the cycle produced by the monument of Yin and Yang which created the five elements. Wood, fire, earth, metal and water. The theory has been used over the centuries to describe the rhythm of nature as she manifested change through the revolving cycles of the seasons. The harvests of plants and seeds. The types of energy nourishing or weakening the organs of the body, astrological evaluation, treatment principles and numerous other correlations to life in general.

It is essential to understand that these elements represented levels of energy. The various levels or frequencies of energy created the organs of the body and this understanding contributed greatly to the development of physiological models. As a medical theory, the five elements were used predominantly to formulate treatment principles. Thus, a working knowledge of the theory was widely implemented in the practice of acupressure, dietetics, massage, herbalism, moxibustion, astrology, and geomancy and exercise therapy.

Yin	Yang
Male	Female
Slow	Fast
Old	Young
Blue	Red
Past	Future
Negative	Positive
Heavy	Light
Cold	Hot
Short	Long
Night	Day
Descending	Ascending
Small	Large
Active	Passive
Direct	Indirect
Action	Reaction
Hard	Soft
Weak	Strong

The relation of Yin/Yang and 5 elements

The elements together with Yin and Yang will determine the state of balance and equilibrium within the body. The five elements as assigned to the organs and bowels are:

	Wood	Fire	Earth	Metal	Water
Yin	Liver	Heart	Spleen	Lung	Kidney
Yang	Gall Bladder	Small Intestine	Stomach	Large Intestine	Bladder

Each organ and bowel are governed by two meridians one flows the left and the other from the right. These pressure points are breathing points for the meridians. There are eight other extraordinary meridians which helps the energy to continue its cycle of circulation, regardless of whether any one of the organs or bowels become decrease and blocks the meridian's circuit. There are other pressure points that cannot be traced to have any connections with meridian.

The law of the five elements

<u>Yin cycle</u>	<u>Yang cycle</u>
Water Destroys Fire (By Extinguishing)	Fire Creates Earth (By Making Ash)
Air (Metal) Destroys Wood (By Cutting)	Earth Creates Metal (By Releasing Gases)
Earth Destroys Water (By Reduction)	Metal Creates Water (By Condensation)
Fire Destroys Air (Metal) (By Melting)	Water Creates Wood (By Nourishing)
Wood Destroys Earth (By Covering)	Wood Creates Fire (By Burning)

Energy flows from one organ to another along five pathways and interacts in the following manner. This information is also mentioned in the book Ninja Death Touch by Ashida Kim, who has gathered the information from his ancestors.

The mother-son law of fine elements therapy

Each element is the "Mother" of the element which follows it along the creative cycle and conversely is the "Son" of the element which proceeds it. Acupuncture never acts directly upon the organ which is diseased – it notifies its mother. If it is too full it notifies Son.

Interaction of the Yin /Yang five elements and organs of Human beings

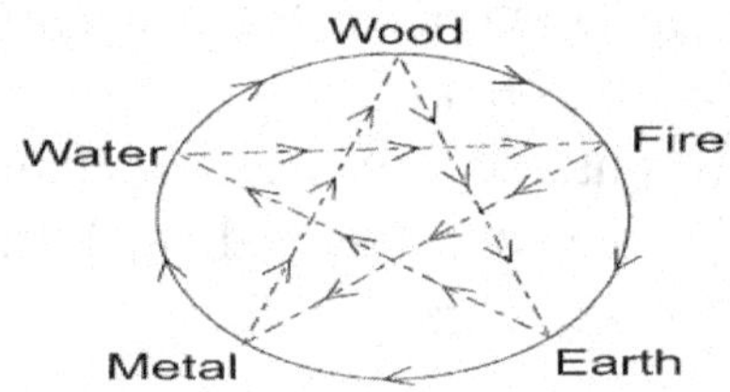

Yang   ——————————

Yin   - - —▸ - - —▸ -- -—▸ -- -▸

The circumference of a Circle represents Yang (Creative) and diagonals of Inner Circle represents the Yin (Destructive).

The above earthly 5 elements and their interactions were believed by our ancestors for the balancing and well-being.

The cycle of Creation (Yang cycle) element creates or produces the succeeding element i.e., fire creates earth, earth creates metal, metal creates water, water creates wood, wood creates fire.

The cycle of Destruction (Yin cycle) element destroy succeeding element i.e., fire destroys metal (by melting), metal destroys wood (by cutting), wood destroys earth (by covering), earth destroys water (by retention) water destroys fire (by extinguishing).

The disease was treated according to these laws of interaction.

Yin for example: Water destroys fire in the Yin cycle (negative) cycle of energy; water is the kidney organ and fire are a Heart organ. So, kidney destroys heart.

Yang for example: Treating the gall bladder, the wood element benefits the heart which is of the fire element (by melting the wood)

Creation Cycle

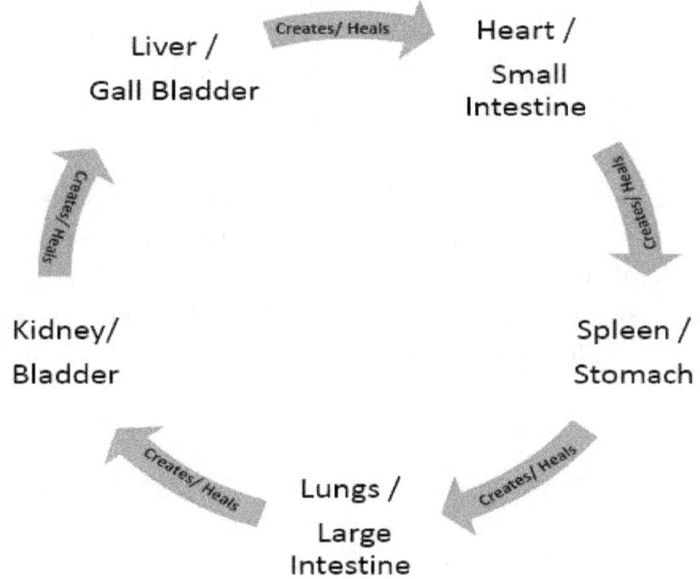

Destruction Cycle

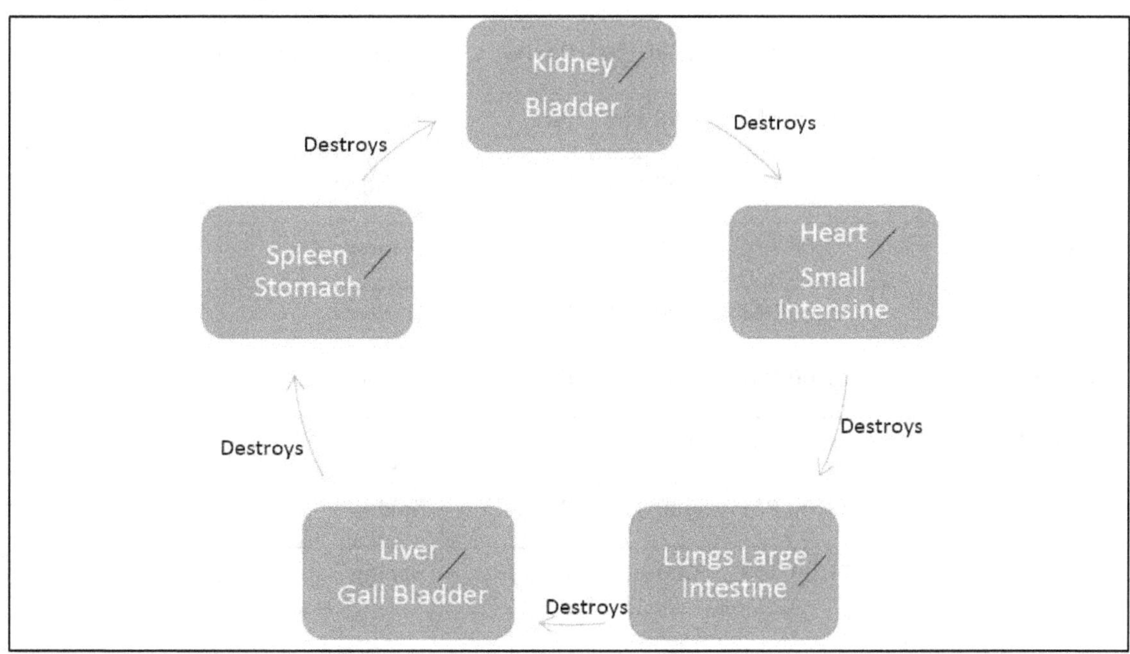

Nei Ching described during 2500BC and Myung Chill King refined element theory on controlling / creative cycle

- Joy (fire element) can be controlled(creative) by fear (water)
- Fear (water) can be controlled by over thinking (earth)
- Worry (earth) can be controlled by anger (wood)
- Sadness (metal) can be controlled by joy (fire).

There are many detailed applications of five element theory to treat or to know about emotions. If the person has liver (wood) problems he is always irritable and angry. If the person has heart fire problems he is in excessive joy. If he has spleen (earth) problem, he always has feeling of any lost and if the person has long (metal) problems he is always sad/ sadness and if the person has kidney (water) problems fear will be predominant.

Organ Timings, Associated element and season

Organ	Timing From	To	Element	Active Season
Lungs	3:00 AM	5:00 AM	Metal	Autumn
Large Intestine	5:00 AM	7:00 AM	Metal	Autumn
Stomach	7:00 AM	9:00 AM	Earth	Indian Summer
Spleen	9:00 AM	11:00 AM	Earth	Indian Summer
Heart	11:00 AM	1:00 PM	Fire	Summer
Small Intestine	1:00 PM	3:00 PM	Fire	Summer
Bladder	3:00 PM	5:00 PM	Water	Winter
Kidney	5:00 PM	7:00 PM	Water	Winter
Pericardium	7:00 PM	9:00 PM	Fire	Summer
Triple Warmer	9:00 PM	11:00 PM	Fire	Summer
Gall Bladder	11:00 PM	1:00 AM	Wood	Spring
Liver	1:00 AM	3:00 AM	Wood	Spring

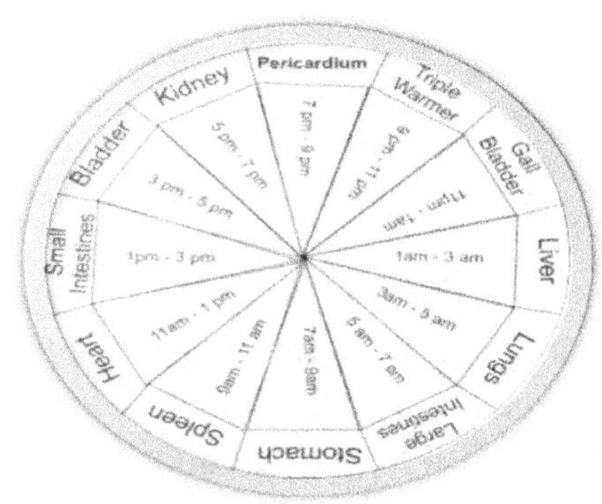

Ancient Indian Mudras

Meditation Mudra

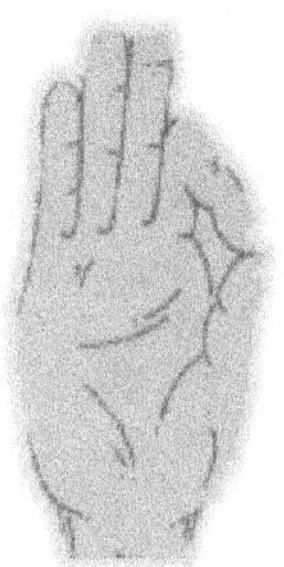

Touch the thumb with index finger pressing lightly

Benefits: This helps in increasing brain power, mental concentration, memory etc. and cures problems of sleeplessness, tension, and lack of concentration.

Vayu mudra (Air)

Keep the index finger on the base of thumb at the mount of Venus and press with thumb as shown in the figure.

Benefits: It cures Rheumatism, Arthritis, Gout, Parkinson's disease and blood circulation defects. For better results, also do Prana Mudra.

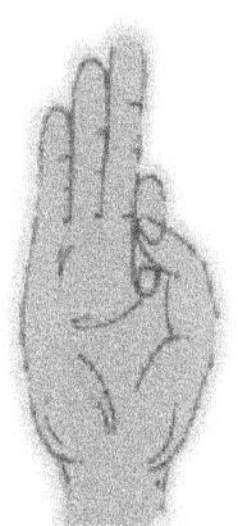

Shunya Mudra (Space) Keep the middle finger at the mount of Venus and press it with thumb as shown in the figure. Benefits: It helps in curing Earache, Deafness, Vertigo etc., It is necessary to do this Mudra for 40 to 60 minutes to get best results.

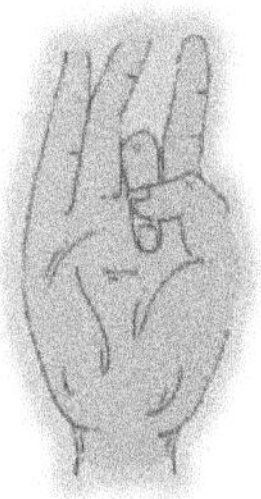

Prithvi Mudra (Earth) Put the ring finger together with thumb as shown in the figure. Benefits: It cures weakness of the body and the mind. It increases life force (Chetna) and gives new vigor to an ailing person. It also gives peace of mind.

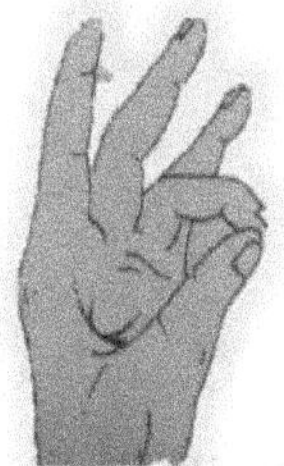

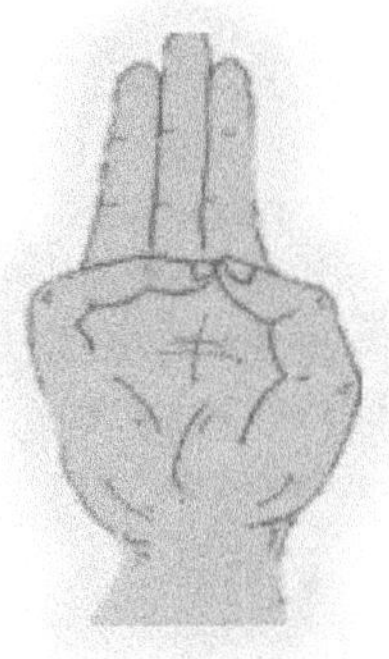

Varun Mudra (Water)

Put the tips of thumb and little anger together as shown in figure
Benefits: It cures impurities of blood, skin problems and makes the skin smooth. Useful in gastro-enteritis and any other disease-causing
dehydration.

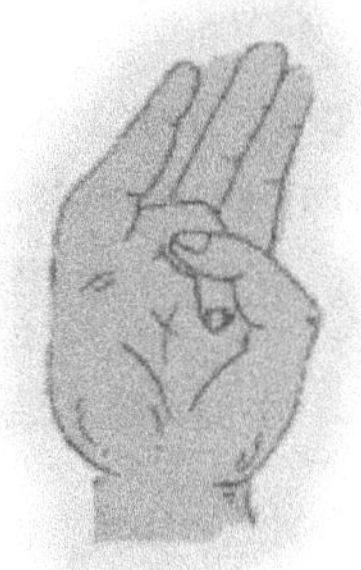

Sun Mudra

Bend the ring finger and on its outer side on second fold.
press with thumb as per the figure.
Benefits: It creates heat in the body, helps digestion and helps in reducing fat in the body.

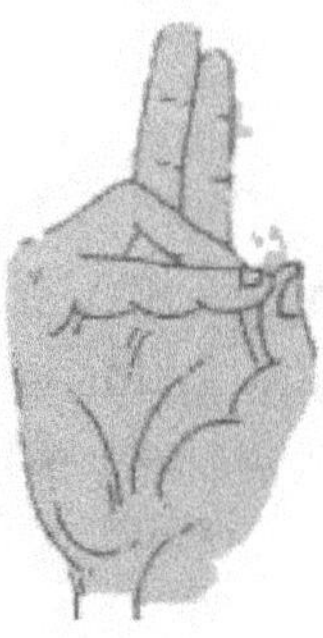

Prana Mudra (Life Energy)

Bend the little and ring fingers so that their tips touch the tip (front edge) of thumb as shown in figure. Benefits: It increases life force and cures nervousness, and fatigue, also helps increasing power of eyes and in reducing the number of glasses.

Ling (Shiv) Mudra

Join both the palms and left hand vertically and thumb of right hand

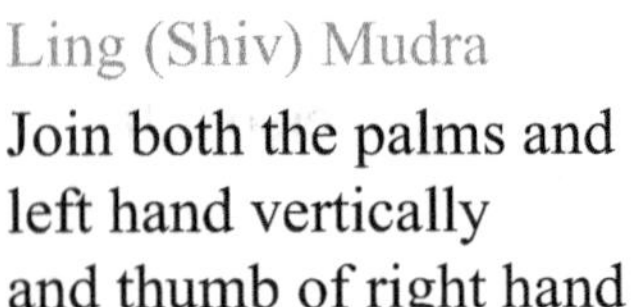
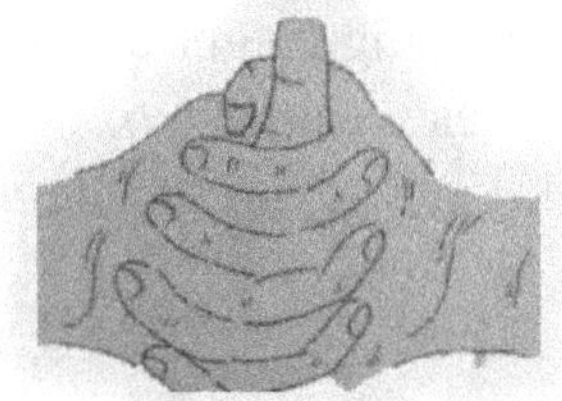

interlock the fingers, keep the thumb of straight and encircle it with index finger as shown in figure

Cancer is said to be the number two killer by Just falling behind heart disease mentioned in the LIZ APPLE GATE and in the Encyclopedia of sports, fitness and Nutrition. As it is well known, it very bitter truth that cancer if not prevented, is very dangerous. Why it considered very dangerous is a well-known fact that the process of cancer is difficult to understand. On the contrary, heart disease can be cured by various medical, fitness exercises and breathing exercises. Hence, let us understand how cancer affects people or how cancer occurs in the human body. Usually, the cells in your body from blood cells to muscle cells grow, divide and die. However, everyday your body confronts a host of carcinogens and substances that can damage your cells. These carcinogens enter your body through the air you breathe, the food you eat and the water you drink. Once it penetrates Inside your body, - the polluted air, water and food may damage cells, altering the cell's DNA (the genetic list of all instructions that guide all activities in our body). Naturally, your body will try to repair damaged DNA but can sometimes fall behind in the unrepaired cell. The set of instructions that tells the cell to stop dividing remains deleted and the cell proliferates dividing out of control, creating more cells with defective DNA. These abnormal cells divide more rapidly and in consequence, they are left to multiply as a result, these abnormal cells begin to squeeze out normal tissue and making it tough for the affected organ to do its Job. Further it affects weaker parts from the cell to organs, but it may depend on the individuals.

Preventive methods
There are many steps to reduce cancer risk, of which the first and foremost is lifestyle habits, and the second one is diet and the last but not the least is exercise. Exercise may help prevent some types of cancers by improving glucose control, which in turn lowers the demand on many organs including your Pancreas. Exercise also speeds bowel transit which means toxins in your waste move through intestines faster. If it is stagnant in the undigested food, there are chances to damage cells in your colon and rectum.

Moreover, Exercise keeps levels of estrogen steady, which may help prevent estrogen related cancers such as breast cancer. For the minimum of at least 45 minutes a day for five days a week is an optimal protection required through various physical and breathing exercises. In addition to exercises, nutrition is also another important factor that could drastically reduce the risk of developing cancer. There are many foods which contain important substances called antioxidants which help to neutralize carcinogens in the body as well as repair damaged cells. The number of research reports on cancer proclaims that optimizing your intake of antioxidant foods (pomegranate fruit) could prevent cancer. You should better avoid artificial and unnatural foods such as fast foods and beverage foods. The other oily fry foods such as potato Chips and French fries may cause cancer. The other important habits of food to be avoided are alcohol, red meat and smoking. Fruits and vegetables contain important antioxidants useful in preventing every type of cancer in the body, and they are also high in fiber which helps to speed up waste transit from the bowel. Hence it is highly and cautiously recommendable for the people, especially in metropolitan cities, to learn to discipline their body with exercise and breathing exercises. Having observed the longevity practices of people from number of countries, I have specially designed some of the most precious techniques both modern and traditional to help people prevent incurable disease like cancer.

I assure that these simple and effective exercises, breathing exercises, and sounds could help people revitalize their body, mind and their spirit as well.

Healthy food for healthy life

"God has a created a natural pharmacy and linked all the needed ingredients for good health" – M. Jayanth Reddy

Eat green leafy vegetables, God given seasonal fruits, beans, peas regularly. These foods contain large number of folate and folate helps to prevent anemia and helps metabolism and maintains new cell creation.

Eating Fish and seafood daily can be very beneficial. Fish contain omega 3 essential fatty acids and they in turn helps in preventing heart attacks. They also improve blood flow to genitals/reproductive system.

Eat Lean meat and white eggs; they contain essential fatty acids, amino acids and a valuable source of protein, essential vitamins and minerals.

For sports persons engaged in strenuous physical activities, follow a high calorie diet. Excess intake of salt not only raises blood pressure but also causes water retention throughout the body.

Follow high fiber diet as fiber is an important food source that improves digestion and helps in nutrients absorption.

Eat warm food all the time. Cold food is not good for the total health because body expects the food to be at the same temperature. Also, warm foods get digested easily and absorbed freely.

Eat B vitamin foods for day to day modern society's problems like stress. Everyone is stress out at one time or another in their life. Many stresses come over money issues, family, kids, jobs, and business. However, the problem is that you will face health problems linked with depression, heart problems, digestion problems, weight gain or weight loss and anxiety. For these problems Vitamin B is the best food to solve above all problems. Vitamin B foods are Almonds, Fish, Whole grains, Pastas, Rice, Milk, Cottage cheese, Cereals, Blueberries.

Eat beetroot, it's very good for the gallbladder and Liver. Also benefits the digestive and lymphatic systems.

Banana contains high potassium and has multi-vitamin, multi minerals with rich fiber. It's an excellent food for muscular system and growing Children.

Blackberries are high in Iron content and are very good for blood deficiency/Hemoglobin/Anemia.

Blueberries helps pancreas and good for diabetic patients.

Carrots, Pumpkin and red Grapes strengthen capillaries.

Yogurt can help fight hypertension.

Coffee can reduce the chance of colon cancer.

Eating Beans help prevent cancer and obesity.

Eating Cauliflower is good for diabetic people and is good for reducing weight, as it contains less calories.

Eat Cherries: They are good blood builders and has good iron content.

Corn is very good for greater bond and muscle build up. It has high phosphorous content and is also excellent food for the brain and nervous system.

Pepper is good for cold, respiratory organs, sinus, ears, bladder, and skin; and good for brain and nervous system.

Eating Cucumber is very good for bowels, skin and keep cool.

Eat Dates as they are very important food for ulcers of stomach and is an excellent food for sports persons who are in strenuous exercise and good source of copper.

Figs are excellent food for arthritis, intestinal track problems.

Eating garlic is good for high blood pressure, and is a remedy for worms, lungs and asthma and all pulmonary infection.

Eat Grapefruit: It's an excellent food for reducing fever from cold and flu. It is also important vitamin for healthy gums and teeth. It's rich in vitamin C and B. Further it also is good for any hardening or body tissues and liver and arteries and good for some cancers.

Eat Guava: Its good for the skeletal and lymphatic system.

Eat Lemon: It's good for throat troubles and cataract. It also helps in digestion.

Eat Mango: They are good for blood cleaner and good for stomach.

Pineapple is good for constipation and digestive. It also has high in vitamin C.

Vitamins and Minerals – Their need and uses

Vitamin A

Vitamin A promotes growth and repairs body tissues, helps bone formation and helps keep the skin and hair healthy. Keeps the eyes function at their best. Proved to prevent cancer and keeps kidney's healthy.

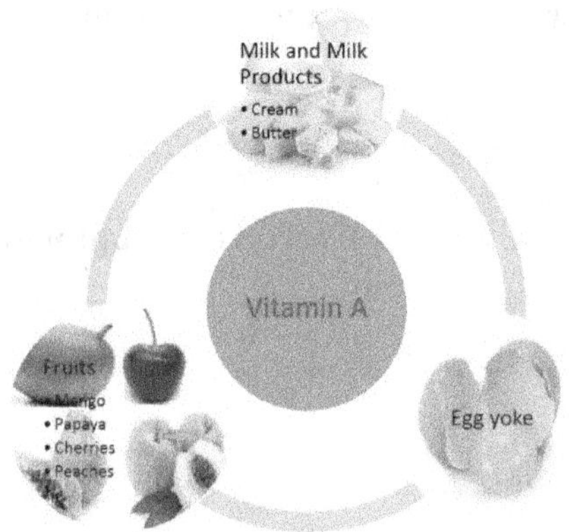

Vitamin is A is available in:

Milk and Milk products (Cream and Butter)
Egg yoke
Mango, Papaya, Cherries, Watermelon, Apricot and peaches.

Vitamin D

Vitamin D promotes/helps build bone mass and helps to maintain blood levels, helps blood clotting, and helps maintain calcium and phosphorous levels. Helps in healthy nervous system and heart functioning.

Foods for Vitamin D

Cheese, Egg Yolks, Milk, Cereals, Animal Liver

Vitamin E

Vitamin E as an antioxidant helps to stabilize and protect the tissues of the Skin, Eyes, Liver, Breast, Testicles, Uterus and protect lungs and red blood cells.

Vitamin E is good for heart diseases, cataract and certain cancers. A known anti-aging agent and helps prevent chronic diseases and is found to decrease cholesterol.

Foods of Vitamin E

Dates, Lime and Oranges, Pudina (Mint) and Methi (Fenugreek)

Vitamin B12

Vitamin B12 is vital for blood formation and healthy nervous system.

B12 deficiency affects the blood, energy levels, and state of mind, nervous system, weakness of arms & legs, looking tired and speaking disabilities

Vitamin C

Vitamin C promotes healthy cell development, wound healing, and it serves as an antioxidant. Also acts as protector against diseases and helps prevent diseases like cancer, cataracts, and heart diseases. Also known to fight against bacteria and viruses

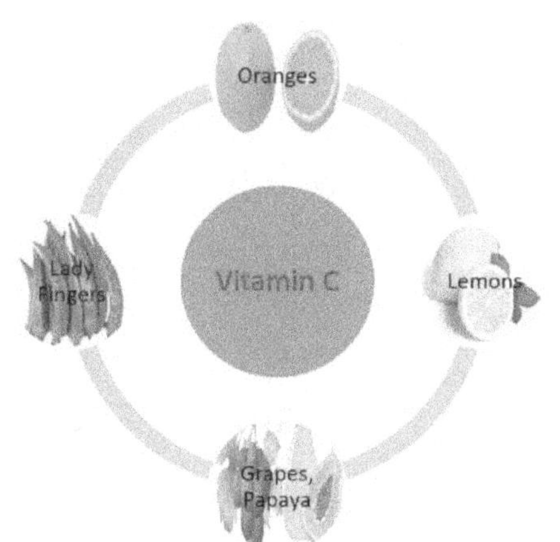

Food for Vitamin C

Oranges

Lemon

Grapes,

Papaya

Strawberries

Dark lady fingers

Calcium

Calcium is essential for development of healthy bones and prevents Osteoporosis. It assists in blood clotting, muscle concentration and nerve transmission.

Foods for Calcium

- Milk, Yogurt and Cheese
- Almonds
- Soya beans Minerals

Copper

Copper will help the body by making the hemoglobin; also carries oxygen to the red blood cells.

Food for Copper mineral

- Nuts - Walnut, Almonds
- Meat
- Seeds o Whole wheat o Dried fruits o Dark leafy vegetables.

Iron

Iron is essential for the formation of hemoglobin, also carries oxygen to the red blood cells and carry oxygen to all tissues of the body

 Foods for Iron

- Dal (Lentil)
- Meat
- Seeds
- Dates

Potassium is one of the most important minerals to protect cardiovascular, nerve functions and for building muscle.

Foods for potassium

- Nuts
- Fruits (Oranges, Banana, Raisins)
- Seeds
- Whole Grains
- Potatoes
- Spinach
- Tomatoes

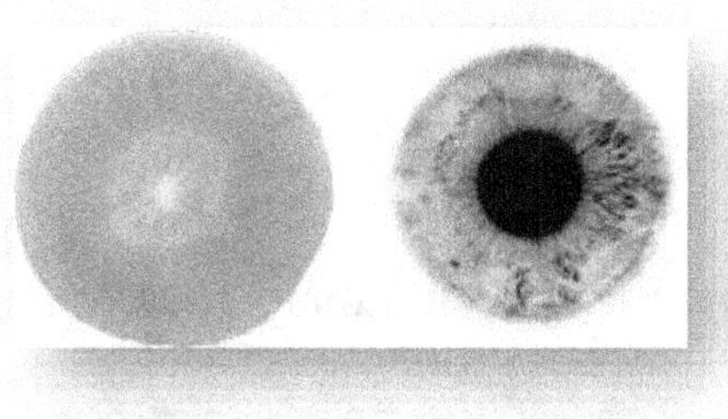

God gave us great clues on what food to eat to keep each organ healthy. I call it 'God's Pharmacy.

Carrot

A sliced carrot looks exactly like a human eye. The pupil, iris and the radiating line looks exactly like a human eye. It's also scientifically proved that eating carrot will keep the eye healthy.

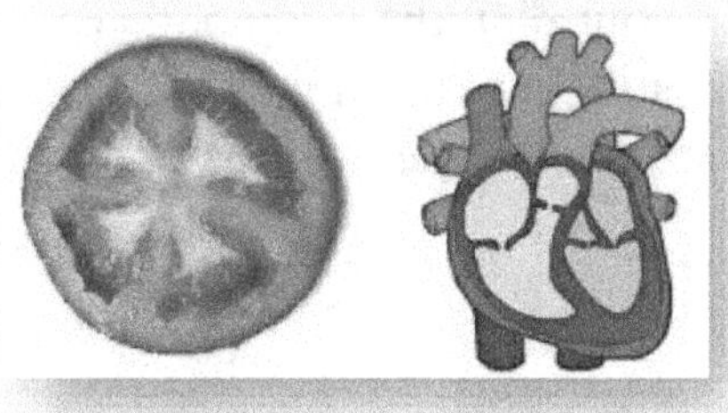

Tomato

A tomato has 4 chambers in red and tomato too has 4 red chambers. Its scientifically proved that Tomato has full of Lycopene, which will help keep heart healthy by purifying.

Grapes

Grapes in hang in clusters just the way heart looks. Each grape looks like a blood cell and even recent researches proved that grapes are great vitalizing food for heart and blood.

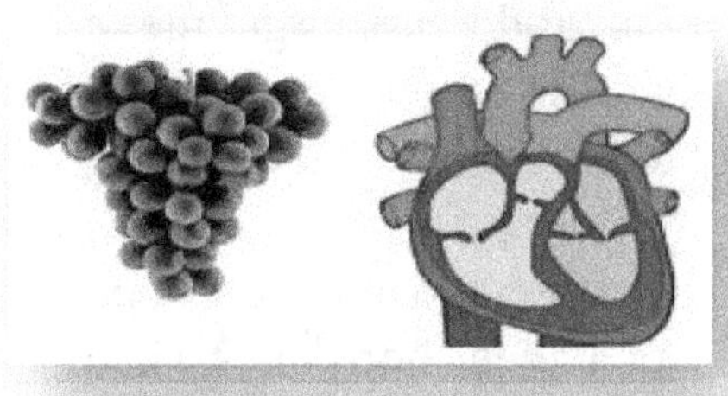

Walnut

A walnut looks like a little brain with left and right hemispheres, upper cerebellum and lower cerebellum. Even the wrinkles and folds on walnut are just like neo cortex of the brain. We now know that each Walnut help develop three dozen neurons transmitters for better brain function.

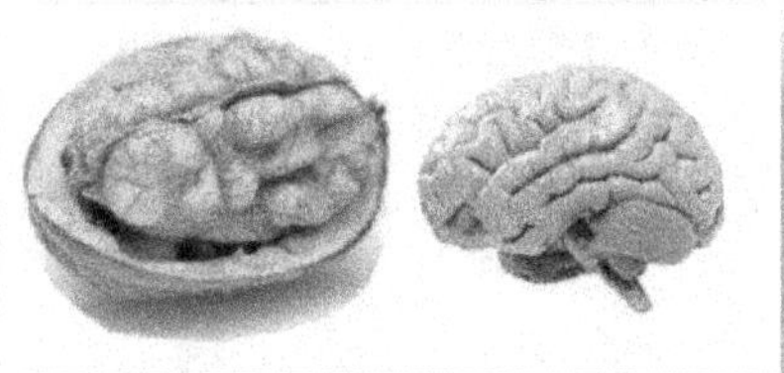

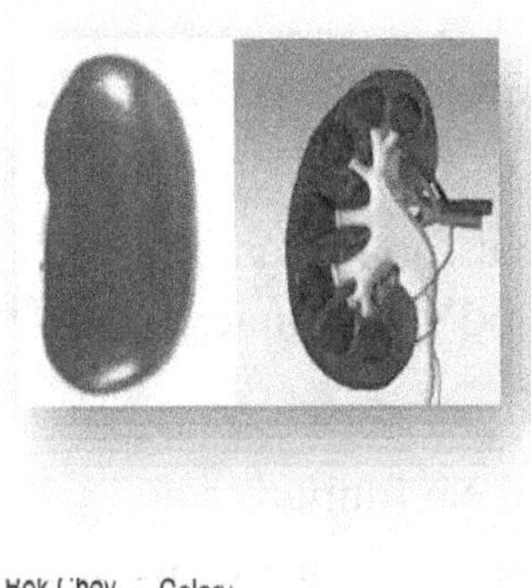

Kidney bean heal and help maintain kidney function; and yes – they look just like kidney

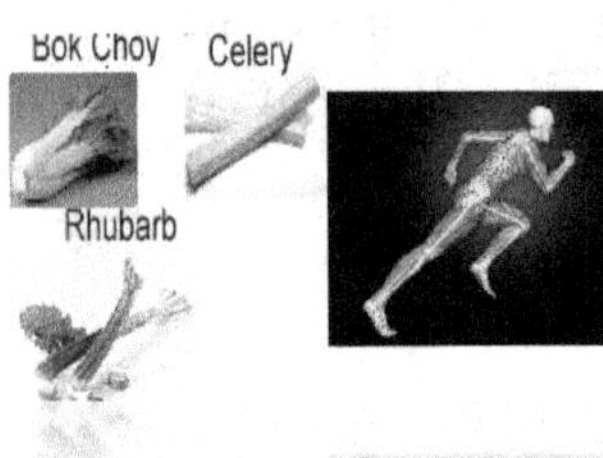

Celery, Bok Choy

Celery, Bok Choy, Rhubarb and many more look just like bones. These foods specifically target bone strength. Bones are 23% sodium and these foods are 23% calcium. If you don't have enough calcium in your diet, the body pulls it from the bones, thus making them weak. These foods replenish the skeletal needs of the body.

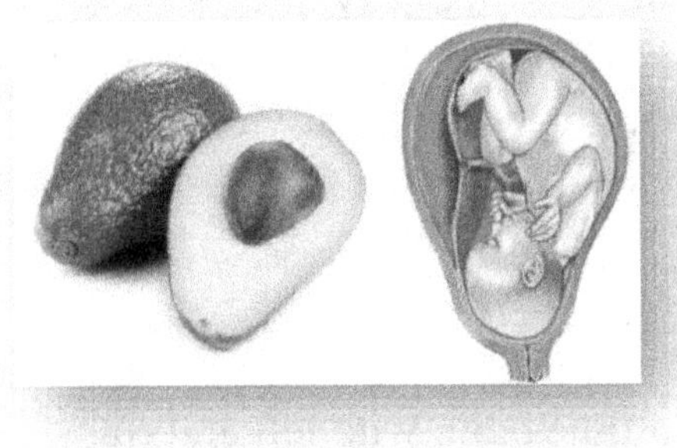

Avocado

Avocadoes, Eggplant and Pears target the health and function of the womb and cervix of the female - they look just like these organs. Today's
research shows that when a woman eats one avocado a week, it balances hormones, sheds unwanted birth weight, and prevents cervical cancers. And how profound is this? It takes exactly nine (9) months to grow an avocado from blossom to ripened fruit. There are over 14,000 photolytic chemical constituents of nutrition in each one of these foods (modern science has only studied and named about 141 of them).

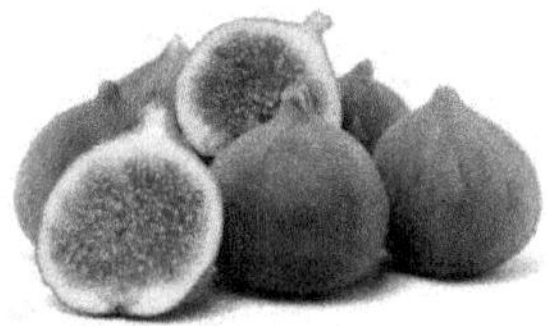

Figs

Figs are full of seeds and hang in twos when they grow. Figs increase the mobility of male sperm and increase the numbers of Sperm as well to overcome male sterility.

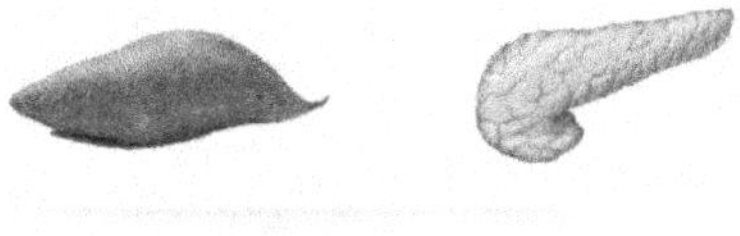

Sweet Potato

Sweet Potatoes look like the pancreas and balance the glycemic index of diabetic

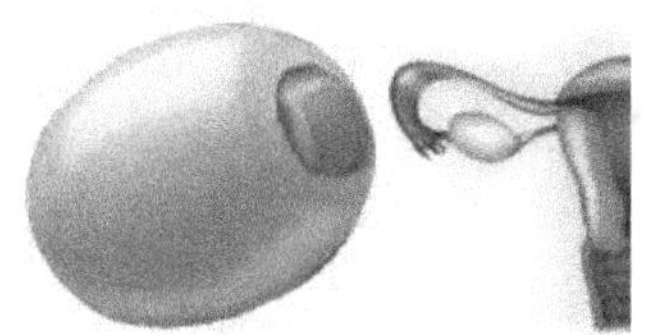

Olives

Olives assist th health and function of the Ovaries

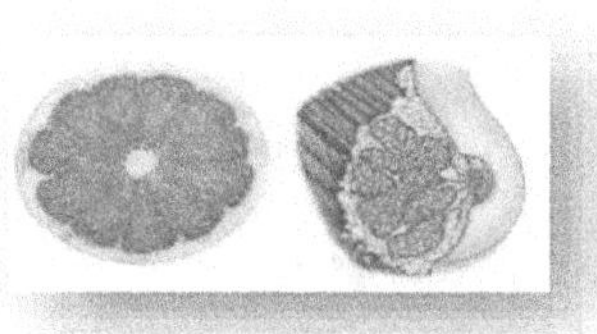

Oranges and Grapefruit

Oranges, Grapefruits, and other Citrus fruits look just like the mammary glands of the female and assist the health of the breasts and the movement of lymph in and out of the breasts.

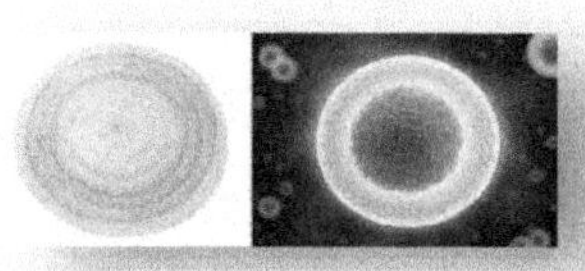

Onions

Onions look like the body's cells. Research shows onions clear waste materials from all the body cells. They even produce tears which wash the epithelial layers of the eyes. Garlic also helps eliminate waste materials and dangerous free radicals from the body.

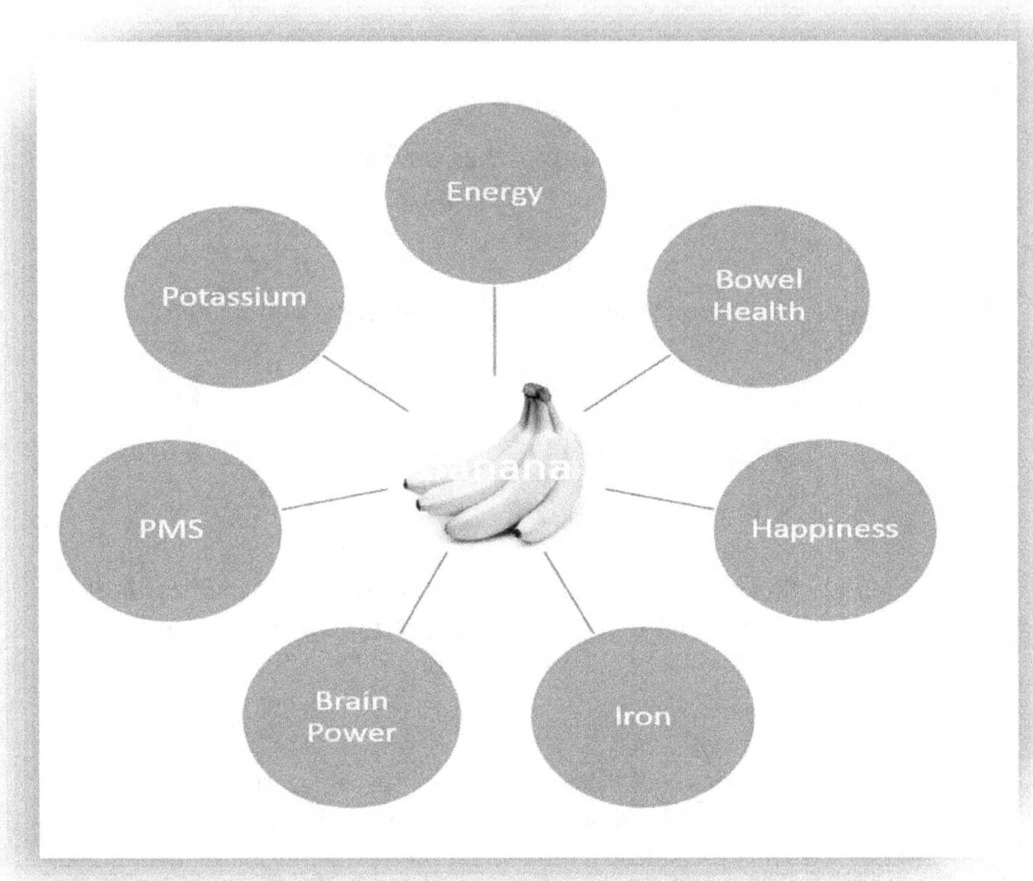

nanas are high in soluble fiber which helps stop constipation and helps to restore and maintain regular bowel function.

Bananas are having high Potassium, which helps deliver oxygen to Brain.

Bananas increases happiness, by releasing a mood regulating hormone 'serotonin'.

Bananas help quit smoking by lessening the effecting of nicotine.

Bananas make the pupils more alert with packed Potassium content.

Introduction to Seasonal Exercises

The basic concept of Season is related to organ – and each organ aligns with the season.

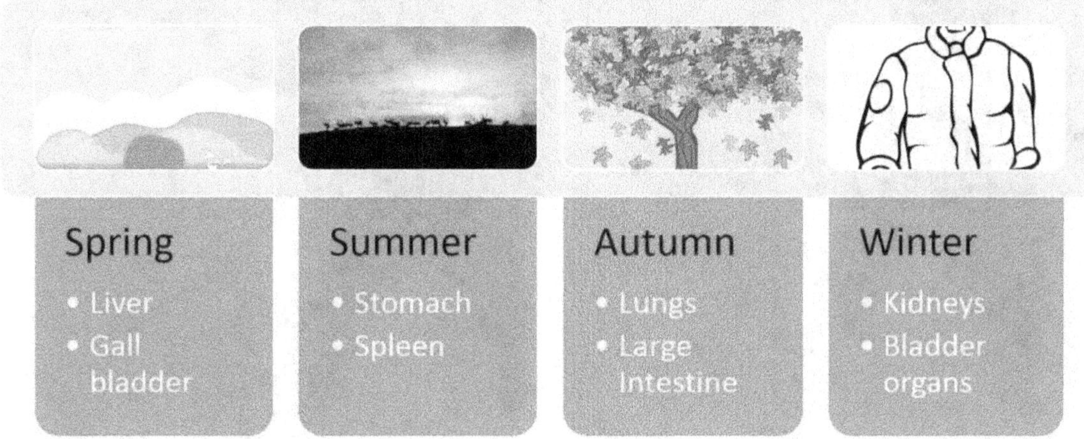

Spring Season and Exercises

Spring is the season for liver and gall bladder organs. So, one must do exercise of meridian points of inner leg, grown, diaphragm, ribs, shoulders and sides of the body during spring to keep the liver and gall bladder healthy.

Horse stance, extend your right hand , twist your left hand at your shoulder, breath out while extending your left hand to the maximum and simultaneously pull your right hand to the hip level – position must be like a bow and arrow. Refer to the Pic1 and Pic2.

Extend your left hand, bend your right hand at your shoulder, breath out while extending your right hand to the maximum and simultaneously pull your left hand to the hip level position must be like a bow and arrow. Refer to the Pic3 and Pic4

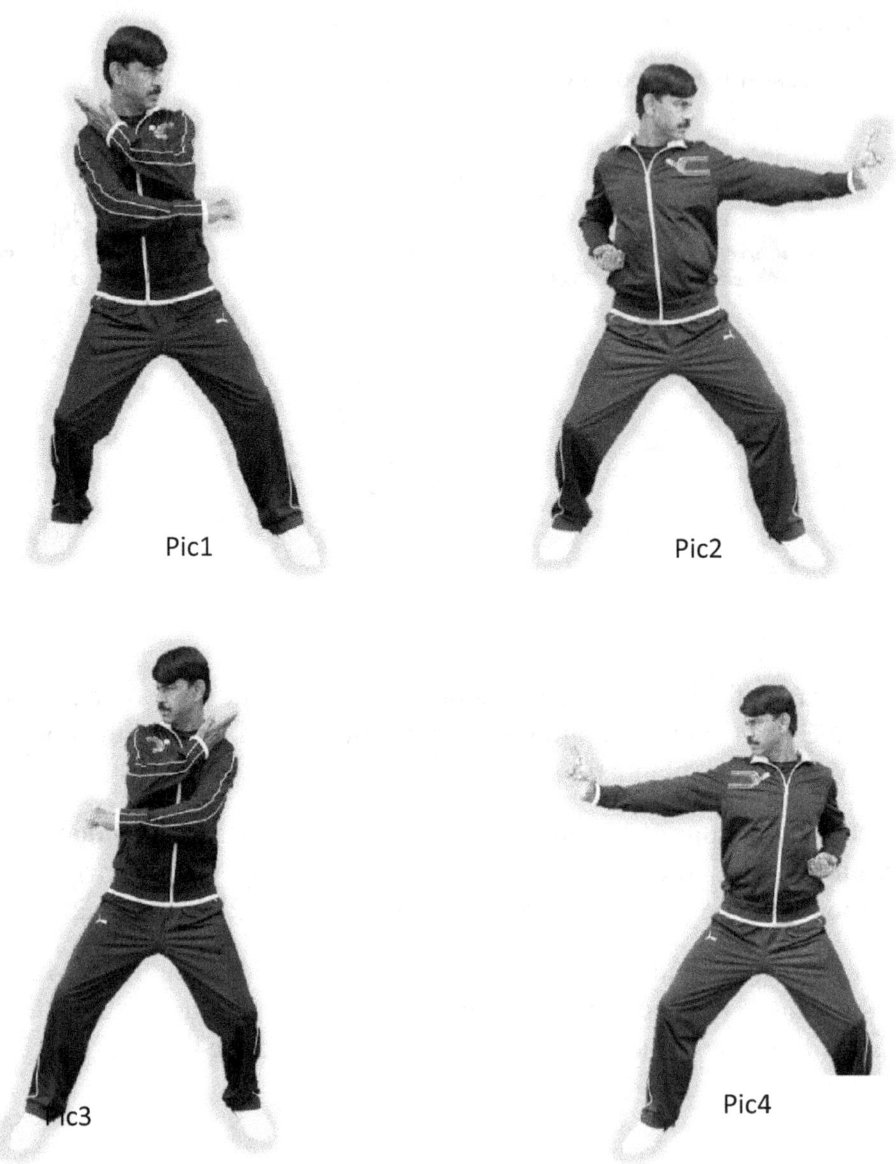

Indian summer

Summer is the season for heart and small intestine organs. So, one must do exercise of meridian points of armpits, inner organs, outer shoulder points, during summer to keep the heart healthy.

Horse stance and extend your left hand with twisting upright of the wrist and turn. Breath in while moving to the other direction. Breath out while extending the other hand like bow and arrow hit, strain your arms.

Breath in with tongue adhered to raft of the mouth and breath out with the lower abdomen. Tongue should be taken out while breathing out.

Stand and extend right palm upwards as if you are holding the sky and press the ground with palm. This should be done simultaneously and feel you are pressing the sky and earth at the same time.

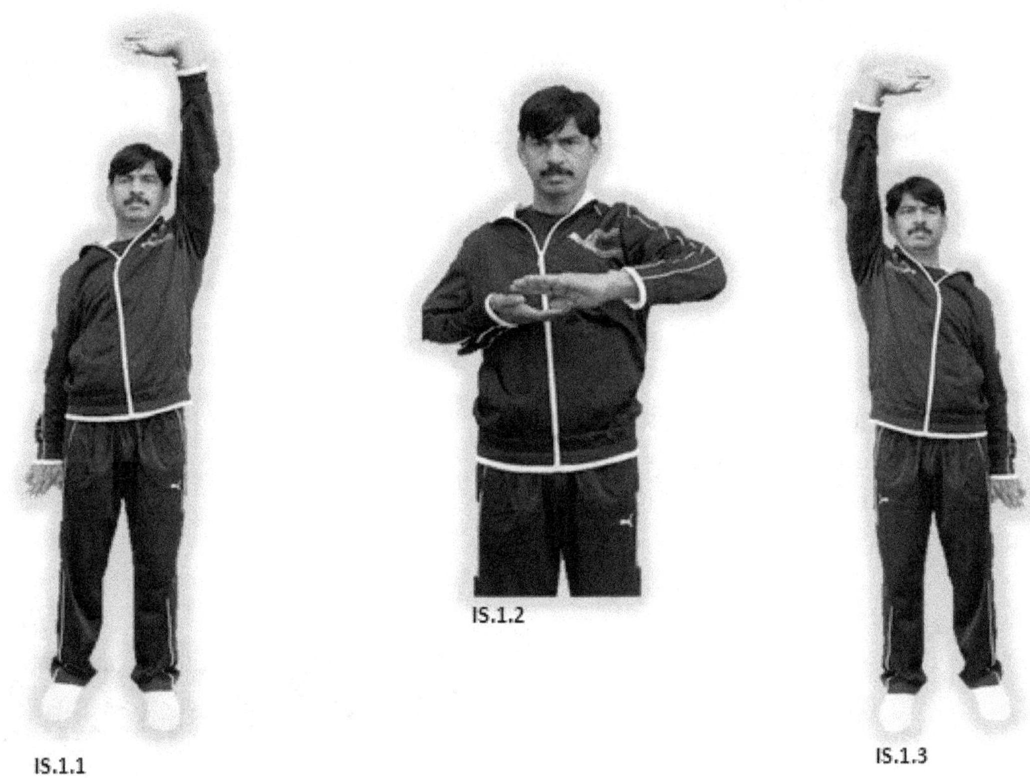

IS.1.1   IS.1.2   IS.1.3

This exercise is advised to be done 6 to 12 times every day. Please refer the pictures 'IS.1.1, IS.1.2 and IS.1.3'

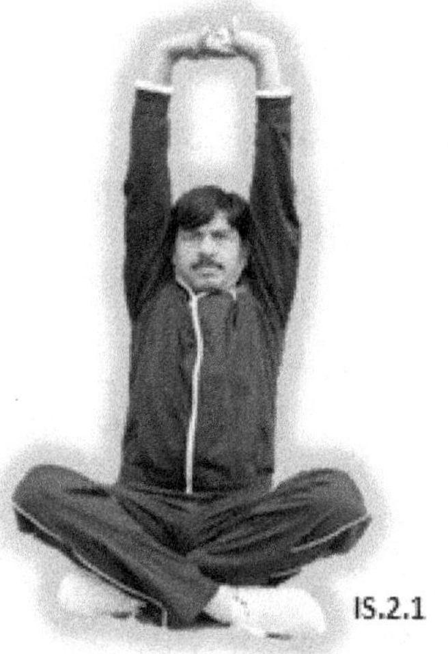

Sit with legs crossed, interlock your hands and pull your hand up as if you are tying a knot. This exercise is good for liver and lungs. Refer the picture 'IS.2.1'

IS.2.1

Sit with legs extended forward; with left leg on the right. Press the leg and change; do 10 times each leg. Refer to the picture 'IS.3.1'

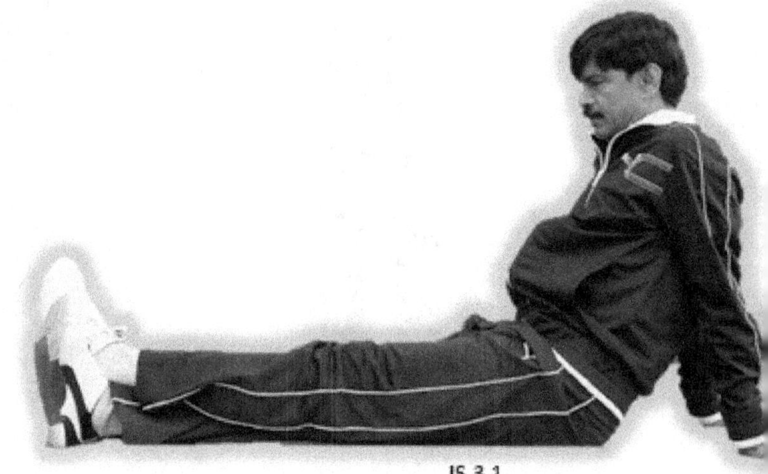

IS.3.1

Autumn

Autumn is the season for lungs and large intestine organs. One must do exercise the meridian points related to these organs during autumn. The meridian points related to Lungs and large intestine are Teeth, sinuses, chest, inner arms and thumbs.

Horse stance and extend your left hand with twisting upright of the wrist and turn. Breath in while moving to the other direction. Breath out while extending the other hand like bow and arrow hit, strain your arms.

Horse stance and punch with the left hand without bending elbow, while slowly breathing out as shown in pictures Pic1 to Pic3; turn to other direction while slowly moving the right hand with breath out and punch slowly see Pic4 to Pic6.

Repeat 6 to 12 times on each side.

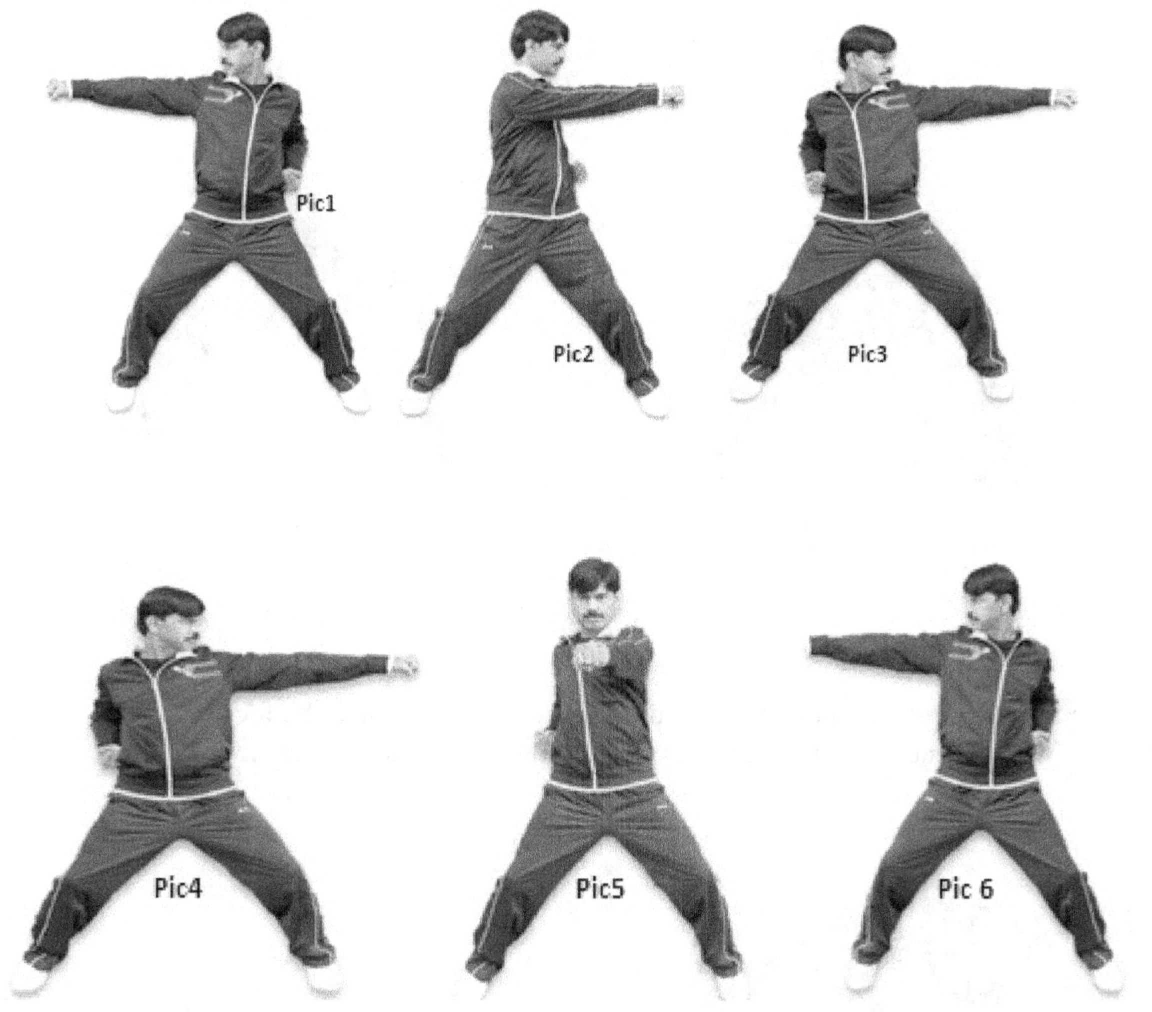

Standing in Horse stance, put your hands on the knees and twist your upper body to the left and always looking straight.

Repeat the same in other direction. Breath-in while twisting to the side and breath-out while coming back to normal position. Repeat the same for 10 times.

Horse stance and extend your left hand with twisting upright of the wrist and turn. Breath in while moving to the other direction. Breath out while extending the other hand like bow and arrow hit, strain your arms.

Refer to the pictures 'A.1 and A.2'.

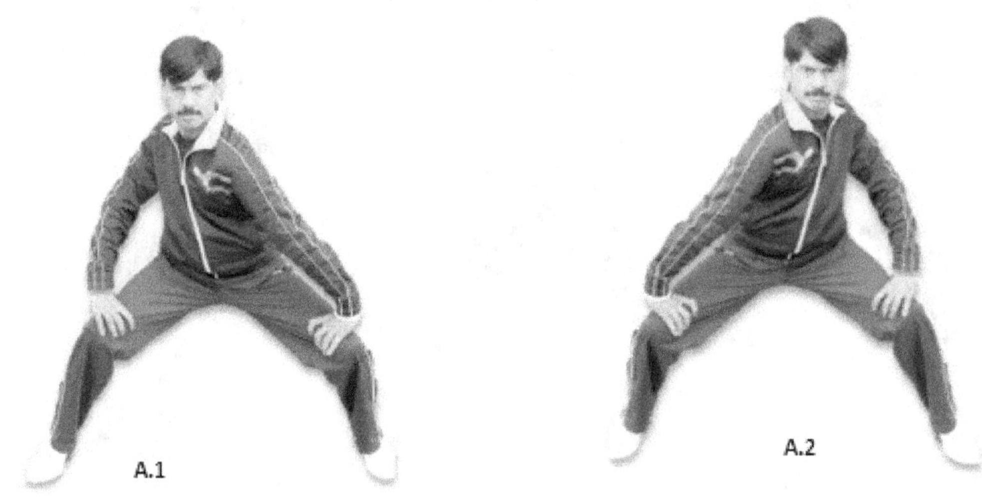

Sit on the ground with legs straight forward and cup your hands to touch the feet with your fingers. Breath in and breath out for 10 times, while holding your toes. Refer to the picture A.3.

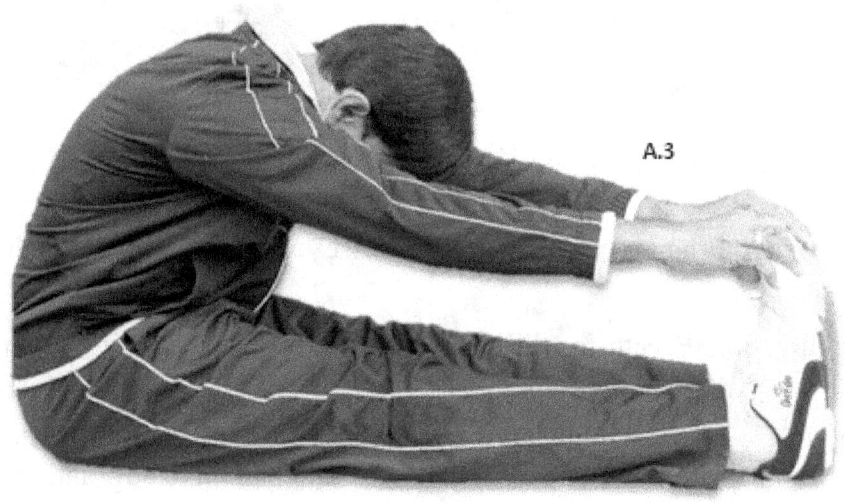

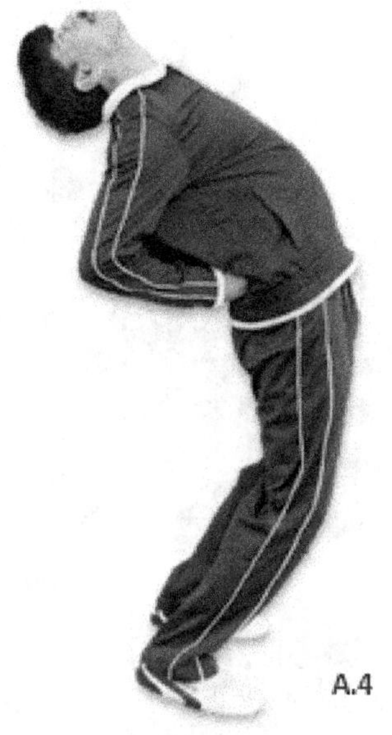

A.4

Stand in horse stance and hand on your hips. Bend back as low as possible. Refer to the picture A.4

Winter

Winter is the season for kidneys and bladder organs. One must do exercise of the meridian points related to these organs to keep them healthy during winter. Meridian points related to kidneys and bladder organs are neck, buttocks, back of the legs, side of the feet, inner legs and chest.

Human body parts are sensitive and weak during these implied seasons and one need to exercise and strengthen these body parts and in return the connecting organ gets impulse and heal or strengthen. Ancient monks and yogis were doing different types of asanas and body movements related to specific meridian points during that specific season and used to solve all the problems.

Sun, Moon and all planets work in a synchronized way and seasons are a result of this interactive synchronized mechanism.

Lie down and touch with nose tip to the knee and be there for 10-30 Second with lower abdomen stiffened.

Repeat the same with another knee.

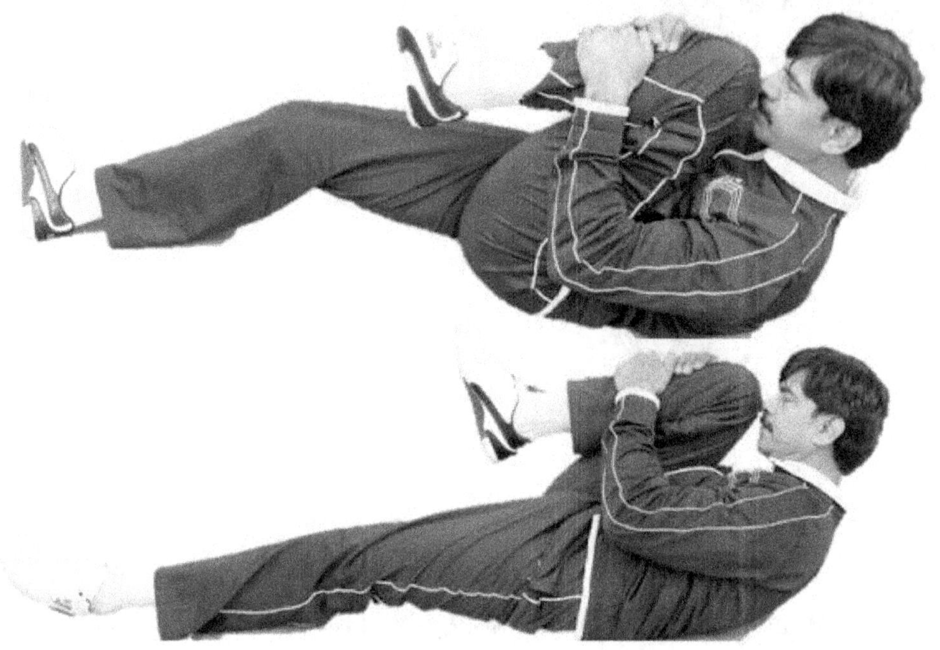

Lie down,
bend your knee
and lift your
lower back to the
maximum and
control;
stiffen your
lower abdomen

Repeat twice the
same for 30 secs
each set

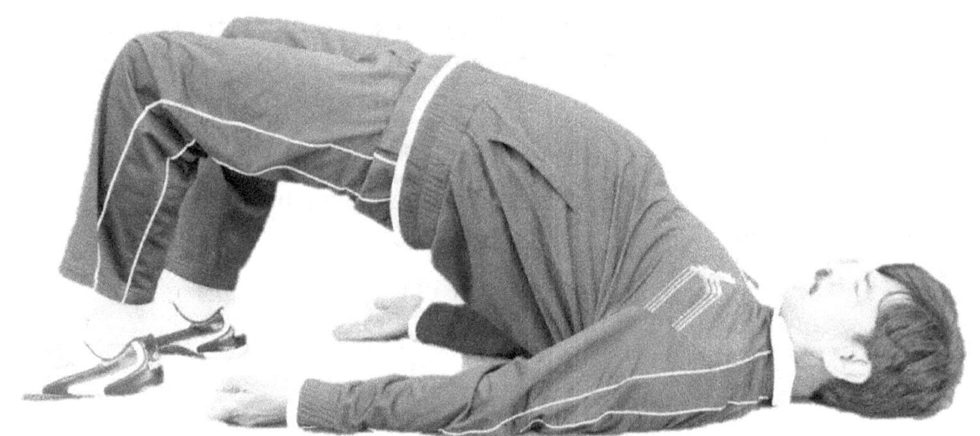

Human body – No need to improve/change

Human body and universe are unchangeable because they are sacred. Human body is perfectly functional as it's the nature of it. We the worldly people are spoiling the health of human body and there are so many methods to correct / improve the spoiled body/health which got unwell due to modern life/modern society.

Today's world is spending time on electronic gadgets/ devise, use motorized transport which are spoiling the human life. Whereas the universe is so sacred, and we learnt many subjects like astronomy, astrology and natural science, but we cannot even alter a bit in the universe or change the way its moving. For example, can we stop the rising sun or Moon or stop the earth from moving? If we even think of it, we are considered mad. We cannot change and moreover, we will be ruined if we try to apply. All we know is the actions of the universe that we face and the symptoms of nature. We don't really know the balance of this world of planets under which we live. We have not even learnt 1% of the knowledge related to the universe and its functioning. Same is the case with human body. We have learned many things about body functioning, but there are lot more uncharted areas.

Further there are billions of starts that are shining in the night which are in in constant motion and they all function in a perfect harmony as one. Similarly, all the living creatures on this planet are to stay in constant motion of the human system in a perfect harmony – since the world and our body contains trillion of cells. There are 12 functional areas namely – digestive, reproductive, lymphatic, excretory, and circulatory, nervous system, urinary system and each of these systems has specific functions and each system interacts with all other systems to achieve and maintain equilibrium in the whole human body.

The present world didn't understand these nature and human body systems. God's ultimate wish is to make every living creature to be happy in every way. We the humans designed to live like birds in the cages, by forming human society. It's incredibly wrong where the human society is lingering with problems like lying, cheating, egoism, selfishness, greedy. Throughout our human existence, societies have built walls and fences to keep others away. Separate races, religions, nationalities, social groups promote prejudices in the hearts and minds of people and create barriers. Hence the human life in the society is constantly in conflict with the self.

We only get one life and we must stop all this nonsense feeling towards other humans. We must build together a beautiful new world of truth and selflessness, there by God will rethink good about mankind and consider his creation is good and not any wrong.

What causes an organ to malfunction?

Modern society creates a life full of physical and emotional stress such as-overcrowding, pollution, radiation with many electronic devices, junk food, chemical additives, anxiety, loneliness, bad postures, sudden or overly vigorous exercise, one or more of the above. These stresses produce tension and start to block the free passage of energy to the body – thus making the organs function defectively. In addition, the concrete jungle that we live in, lacks the safety valves provided by nature - like trees, open spaces with fresh air and thus impacting the organs. The question that arises is that of our activities disturb the natural process or mechanisms of preserving health. The matter requires our serious attention.

Vital Organs – Functions, causes of disease and keeping them healthy

Human Heart

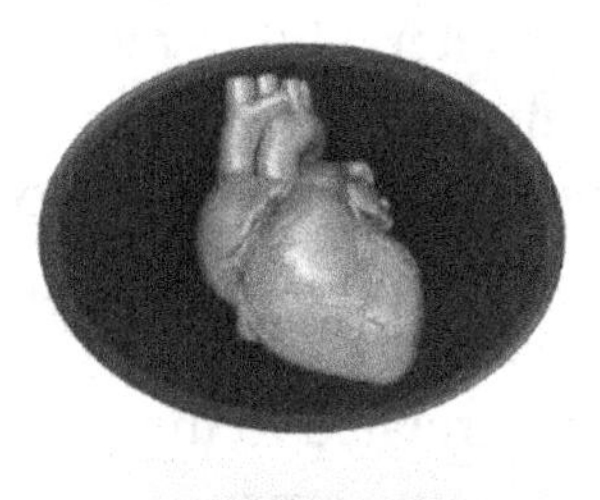

Key functions of heart

Human heart is a vital organ that Pumps the blood through the body via circulatory system and supplies oxygen and Nutrients to the tissues. It also removes Carbon Dioxide and other waste.

Heart Weight is roughly 280gm to 340gms (Male) & 230gms to 280gms (Female). It beats 60 to 80 times per minute and pumps 5 to 6 liters of blood throughout the body.

Mental functions of thinking, memory and concentration as well as sleep and dreams depend open a health heart.

Causes of Heart diseases

Below image depicts the primary risk categories for heart.

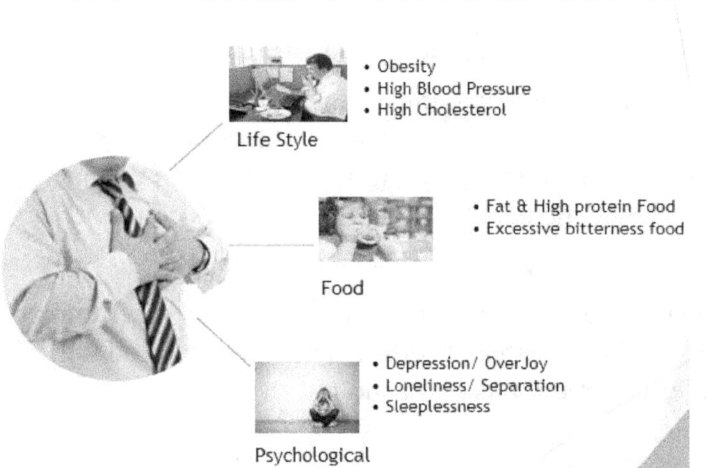

Type of lifestyle has huge impact on the health of heart. Sedentary life style will directly impact the blood pressure and cholesterol.

Second most important factor impacting the heart's health is food. High fat and high protein food will impact the heart's function. Also eating excessive bitterness food will take a toll on heart.

Another important set of factors that will impact heart are emotional and psychological.
Depression or over joy, Loneliness or separation, sleeplessness will make the heart weak.

People with heart problem will not be in good health during summer (heat).

For a healthy heart

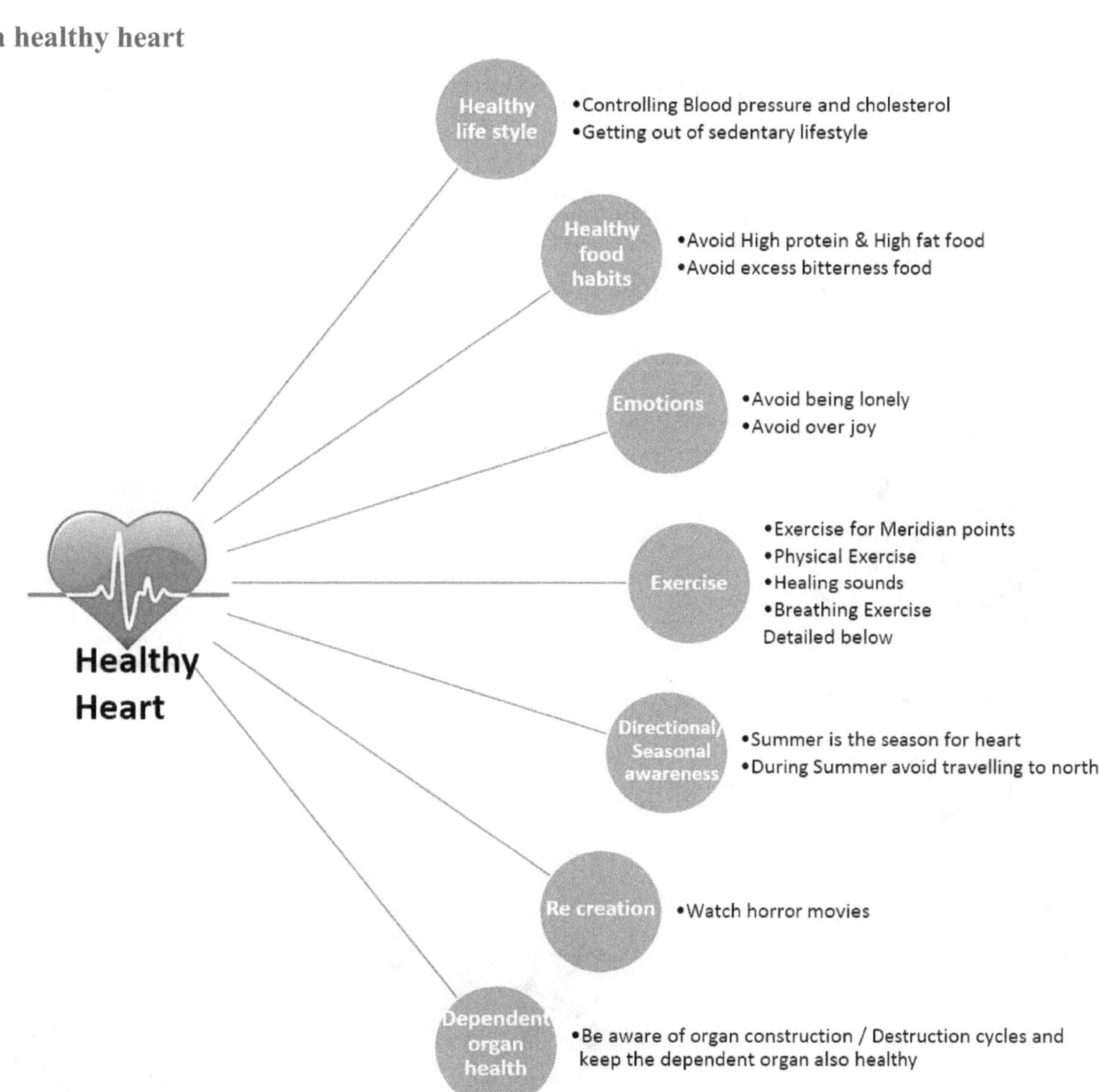

If a person is diagnosed with any heart related ailment, one must.

- Follow a healthy lifestyle, keep checking the cholesterol and blood pressure levels every 3 months.
- One must avoid taking high protein and high fat food till he ailment is brought to control.
- One must avoid being lonely and should avoid over joy.
- Must get involved in exercises that are prescribed (Meridian points, Physical, Breathing techniques and Healing sounds).
- One must also not travel to northern part of India, as its relatively hotter during summer.
- Should start watching Horror movies.
- Should also keep the dependent organ (Stomach/Spleen & Lung/Large Intestine) in good health.

Symptoms of heart ailments

Palpitations, depression, mental problems like anxiety, nervous system disorder like neuro-dermatitis.

Exercise for heart

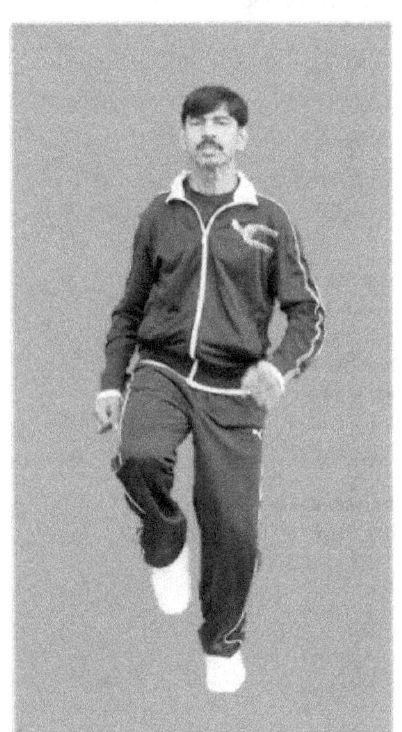

Running on the spot for 1 minute continuously, with knee lifting at the hip level; will immensely benefit heart.

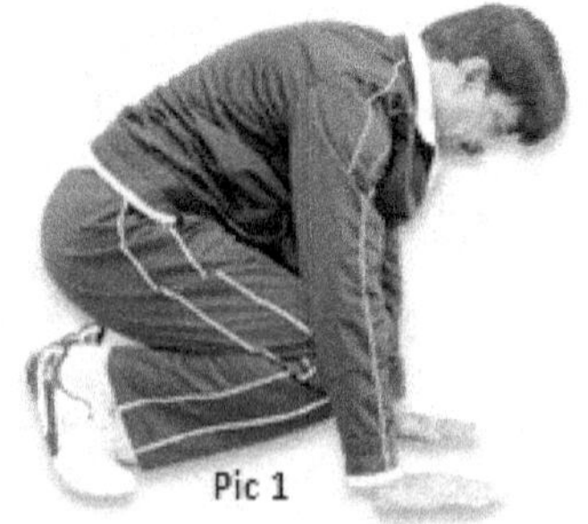

Pic 1

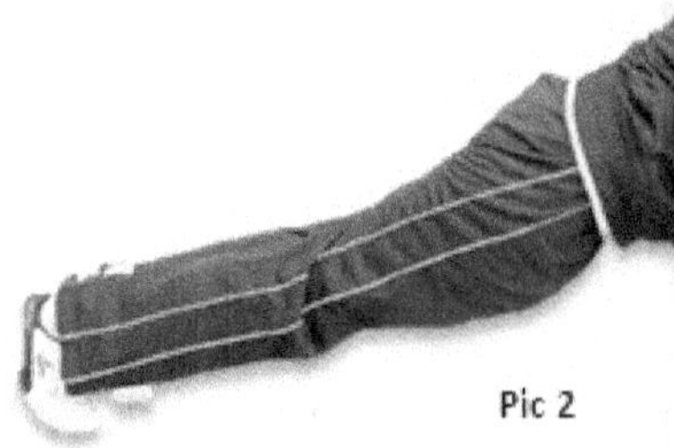

Pic 2

It is recommended to do the Cardio exercise as shown in the picture above – with palms on the ground, bring your knees near to the hands. Keep going back and forth, as shown in the pictures above.

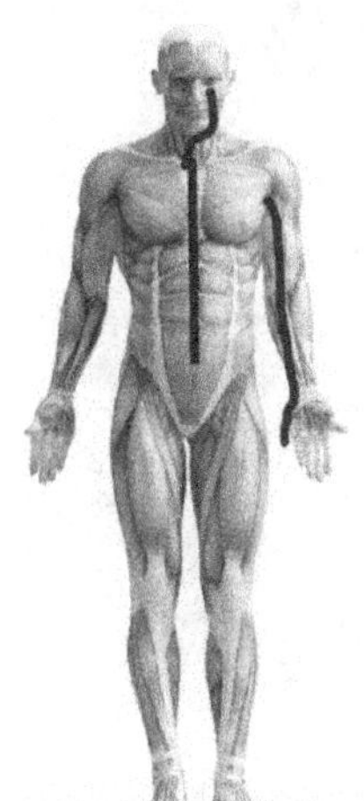

Exercising these points will help getting rid of all heart related problems.

Heart meridian points runs from heart, armpit externally along the medial side of the arm elbows to inside of the little finger.

The other points also run from diaphragm connected with the small intestine; also points runs from throat to eyes.

Exercising these points will help getting rid of all heart related problems.

Heart Meridian Exercises

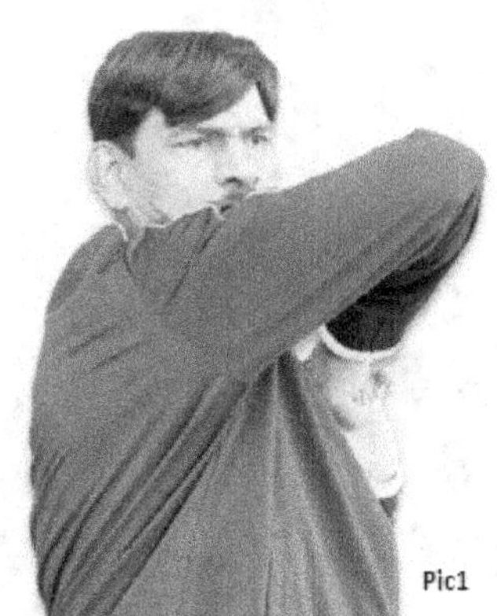

Pic1

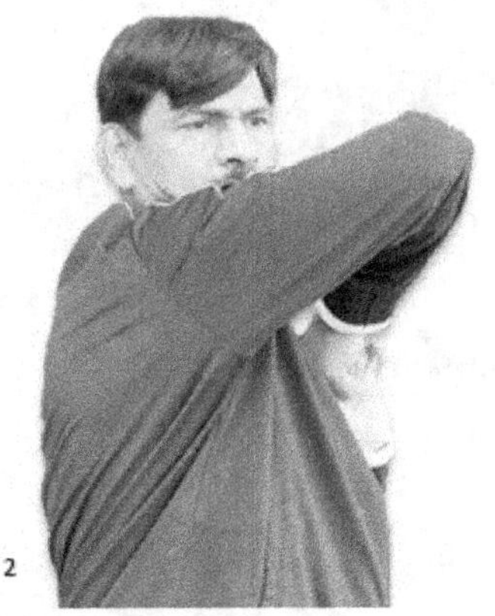

Pic 2

Holding the knuckle with palm of the hand and hit elbow to face with left hand and right hand

Horse stance with palms facing upwards and push the palms to the sideways while locking the elbows and while breathing out. Breath in and bring the hands to the hip level. See pic 1 and 2

Horse stance and push your palms straight sideways without bending and while breathing out.

Breath in with hands at hips and breath out while moving hands over the head, without bending elbows.

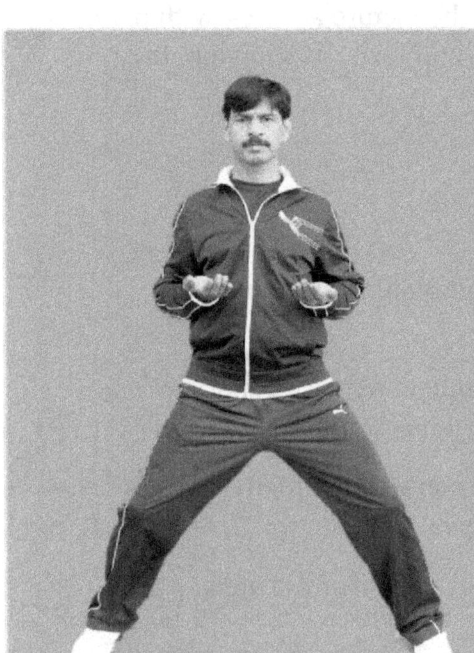

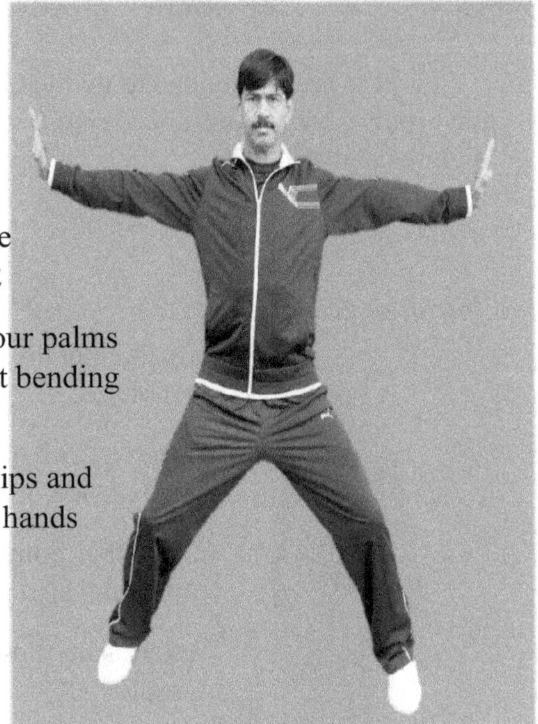

Spread your legs in horse stance with knees bent with double shoulder width between knees, and open hands at the hips, breath in and breath out while moving the hands straight to the chest level. Refer to the pictures. Repeat this for 50 times.

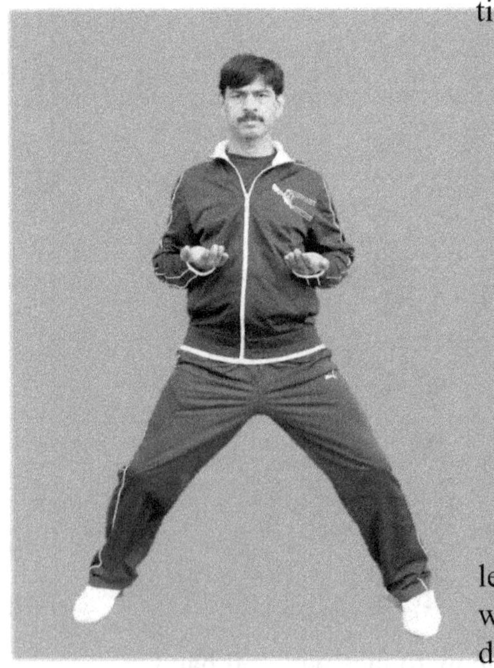

Spread your legs in horse stance with knees bent with double shoulder width between knees, and open hands at the hips, breath in and breath out while moving the hands straight to the chest level. Refer to the pictures. Repeat this for 50 times.

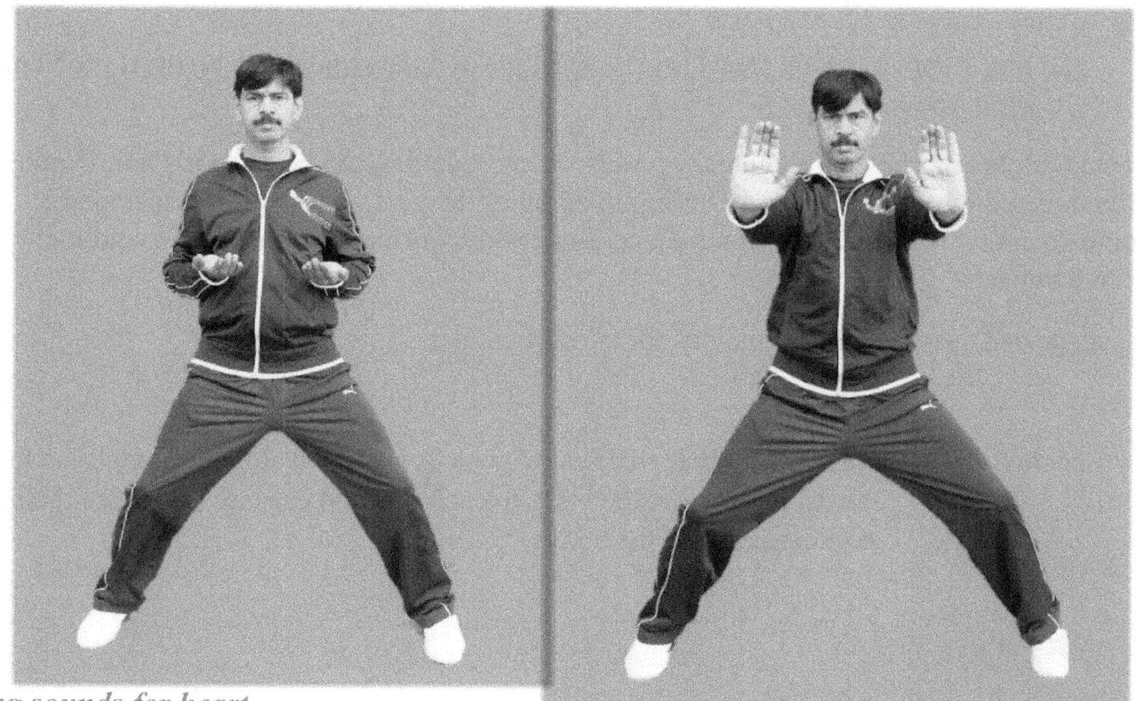

Sit on chair with hands interlocked with hands bent to the right side, so that left ribs and chest contracts and do the sound below mentioned. Bring back the hands to the lap each time and imagine heart in red color and feel it and continue for at least 12 times daily.

Heart Sound is HAWWWWWWWWW or HAAAAAAAA or HAUUUUUUU. It is recommended to make this sound at the prescribed timing, which is between 11AM and 1PM. Heart is sensitive during the summer season.

It is recommended to do this exercise in front of a Peepal tree, for immediate results. It's difficult to grow Peepal tree in India at everyplace. According to Indian Ayurveda, Neem tree is also best to do breathing or any sounds. Doing breathing and sounds exercises under Neem tree will improve and help get quicker results. But if you do not have neither of the above, you can practices breathing and sounds under any tree which gives oxygen.

Breath in with tongue adhered to raft of the mouth and breath out with the lower abdomen. Tongue should be taken out while breathing out.

During summer season Heart is very sensitive and many people with heart problems are not in good health.

People with heart problems shouldn't go to Northern side of India because it's hot. People are easily angered during this season. During this time of the year, mass murders take place, people go crazy. It's preferred for people to go to South during this season, to avoid the adverse impacts.

It is suggested to watch Horror movies for a healthy heart.

Human Lungs

Key Functions of the lungs, the air that we breathe goes to the blood stream through the lungs and carried throughout the body to each cell and organs. Lungs are the hardest working organ in the body.

Causes of Lung diseases

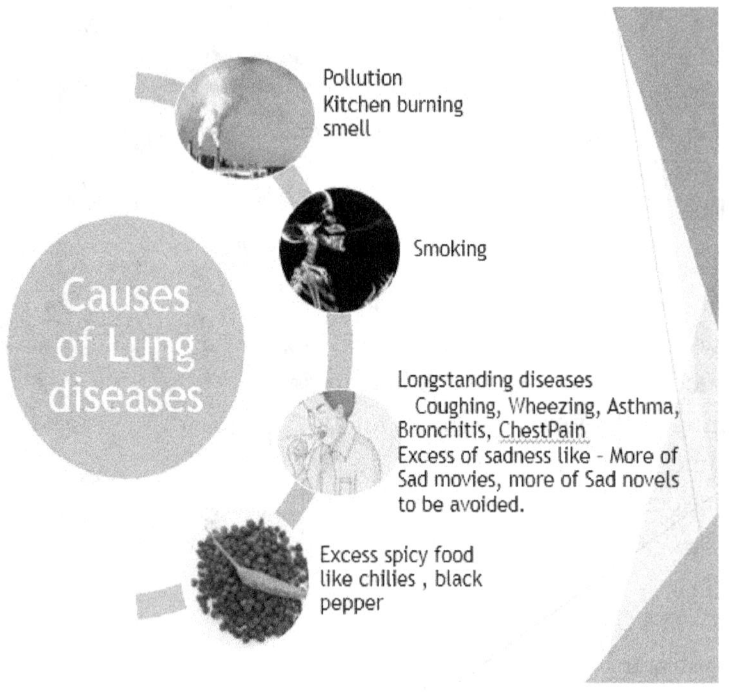

Environment plays a crucial role in keeping the lungs healthy. Pollution, burning smells from Kitchen will prone the lungs to diseases.

Smoking makes the lungs choke and reduces the longevity of the lungs.

Any lung related longstanding illness will take a toll on the health of lung.

Also eating excess spicy food will impact the lungs directly.

People facing chronic illness like wheezing, asthma, chest pain leads to lung diseases/cancer.

Chronic sadness will lead to deficiency of lung. Avoid Sad atmosphere, avoid watching sad movie.

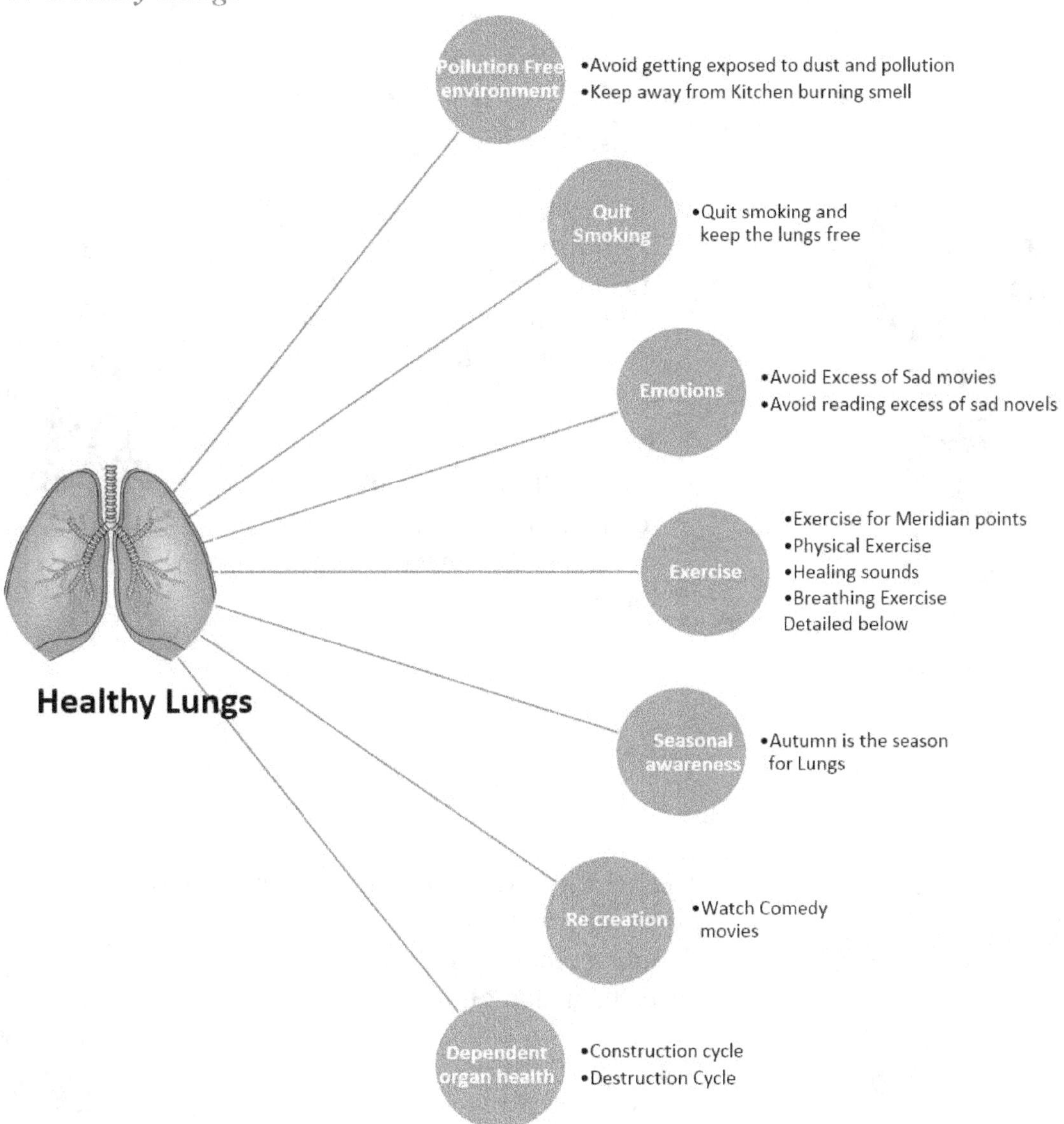

If a person is diagnosed with any type of lung disease, he should

- Avoid getting exposed to dust and pollution. Must keep away from kitchen and other burning smell.
- Immediately quit smoking.
- Avoid excess sadness; avoid sad movies and stop reading sad novels.
- Watch comedy movies/shows and read comics.
- Make sure that the associated organ in the construction cycle is taken care.

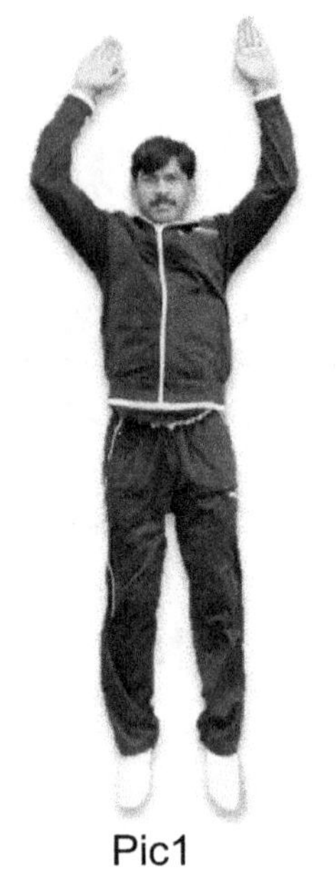

Pic1

Jumping and Volleyball hit for 20 times(as shown in Pic1) and jogging for 30 mins (See pic 2) daily will keep the lungs in good condition.

These all exercise will impact on internal stimuli on cells, tissues and connecting lung organs.

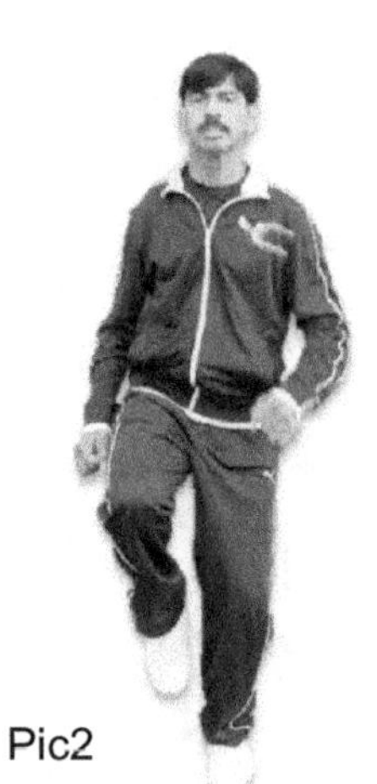

Pic2

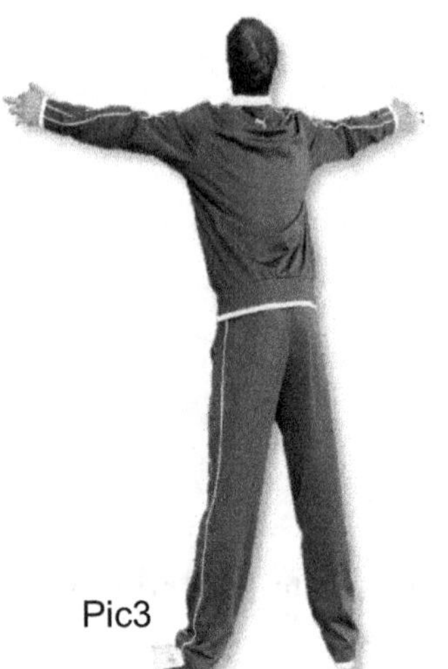

Pic3

Keep 3 feet away from the wall and lean on – keep stretching hand straight without bending elbows and breathe in. Breathe in and out for 10 times.

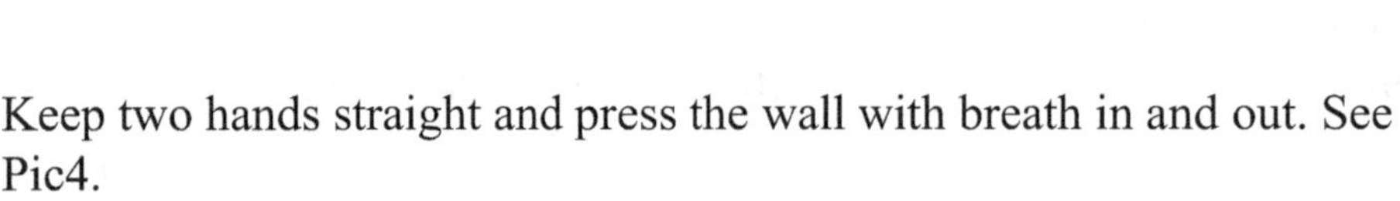

Pic4

Keep two hands straight and press the wall with breath in and out. See Pic4.

Maintain 3 feet distance from the wall.

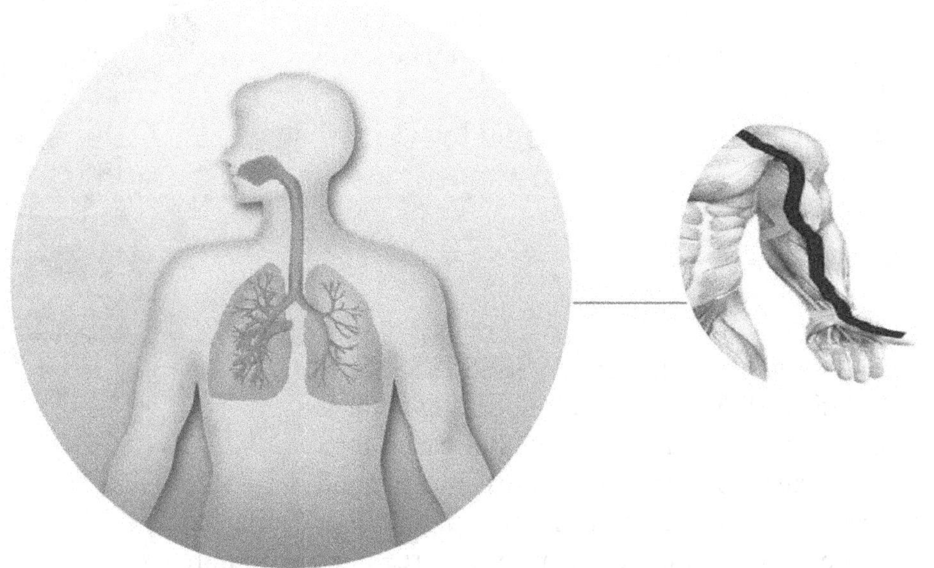

These points and connected muscles if we exercise and pressurize the points of these meridian, can help problems of breath, sore throat, sore arm and lungs overall.

Lung Meridian Exercise

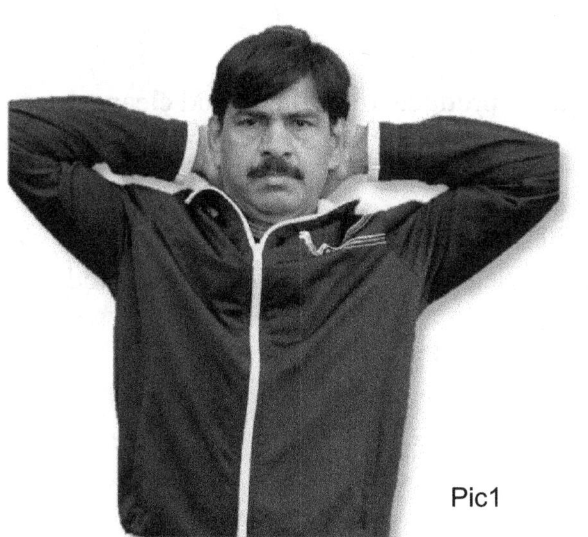

Pic1

Stand and interlock hands behind your neck and press hard for 10 seconds. Repeat for 10 times.
See Pic 1

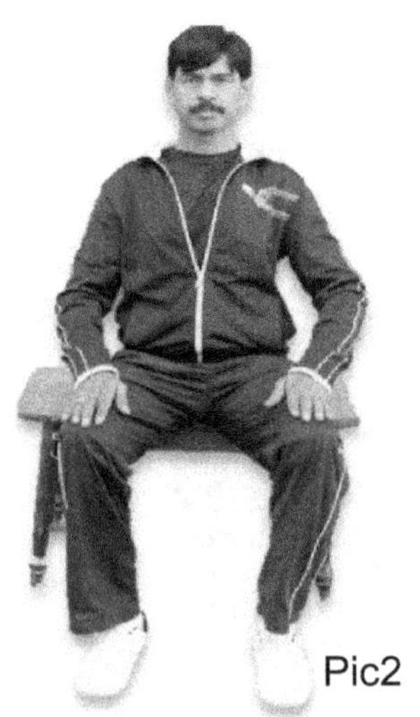

Pic2

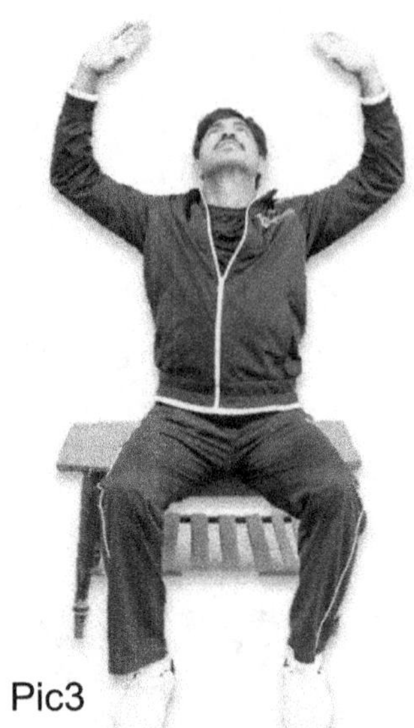

Pic3

Sit on a chair with hand bent at the elbows as round above the head (as shown in Pic2 and Pic3) and give sound below mentioned
HISSSSS
each time you do visualize your Lungs in white color.

Lung Sound is HISSSSSSSSSSSSSSSSSS or THSSSSSSS and the nature of Lung color is white. Timing of lungs is between 3 am to 5 am and the season for Lung is Autumn. Doing this exercise in front of cypress tree is good and will get immediate results. You can do in front of mango tree or Tamarind tree as well. If you are not near to these trees, one should do this near any tree/plant with pure oxygen.

Kidneys

Key functions of kidneys

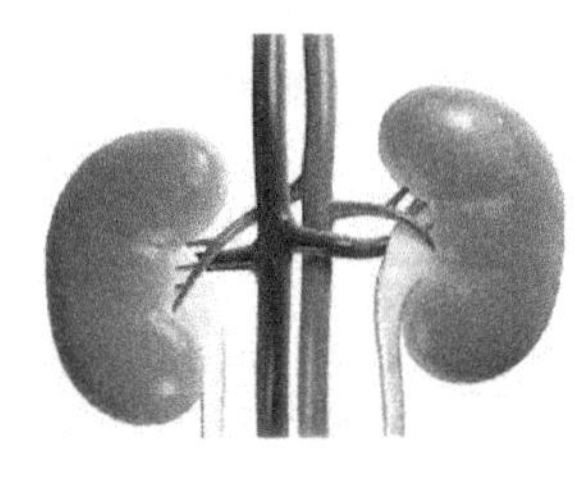

shortening of breath

Kidneys help filter waster products from blood and cleans the blood – removes excess fluids thereby maintaining balance of salt and minerals.

When kidneys stop filtering the blood/removing the waste – causes swelling in ankles/legs/body, vomiting sensation and

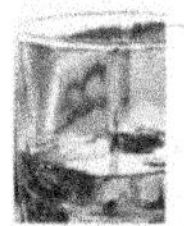

Causes of Kidney Problems

Excess intake of liquor

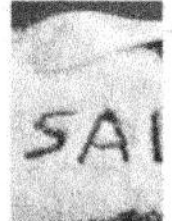

Excess salt

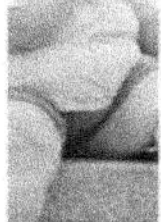

Lack of exercise

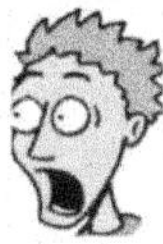

Emotions like fear

Excess intake of liquor and more than normal intake of salt will destroy the kidneys. Lack of exercise and emotions like fear will keep the kidneys prone to ailments.

For Healthy kidneys

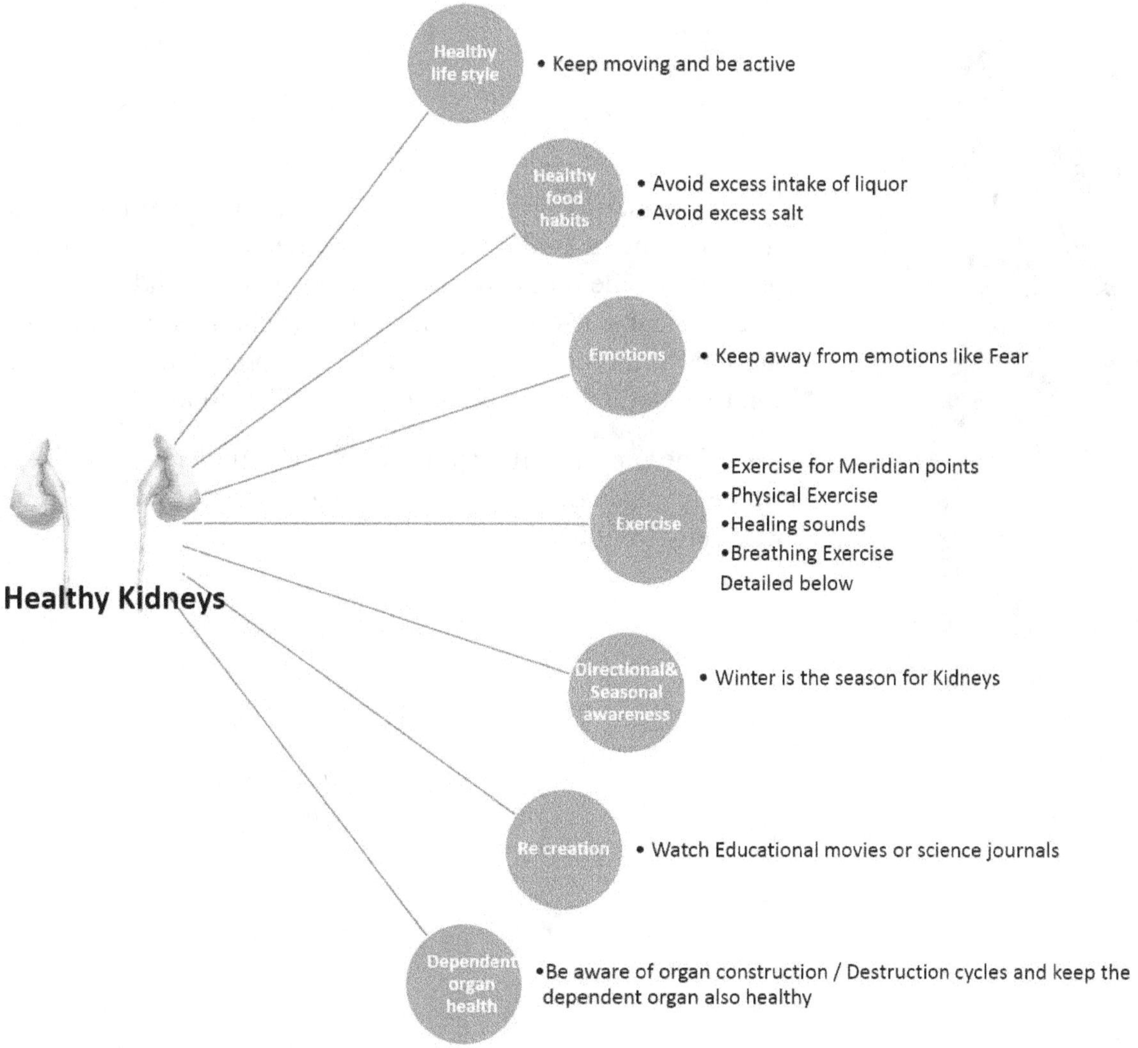

Healthy life style
• Keep moving and be active
Healthy food habits
• Avoid excess intake of liquor
• Avoid excess salt
Emotions
• Keep away from emotions like Fear
Exercise
•Exercise for Meridian points
•Physical Exercise
•Healing sounds
•Breathing Exercise
Detailed below
Directional& Seasonal awareness
• Winter is the season for Kidneys
Re creation
• Watch Educational movies or science journals
Dependent organ health
•Be aware of organ construction / Destruction cycles and keep the dependent organ also healthy
Healthy Kidneys

If a person is diagnosed with any kidney related ailment:

- He must be active and moving, instead of sedentary.
- He must avoid excess intake of liquor.
- He must reduce the salt intake.
- He must keep away from emotions like Fear/depressed.
- He must be more careful during winter.
- He must watch Educational movies and read science journals.
- He also must take care of associated organ in construction/destruction cycle.

Meridian Points for Kidneys

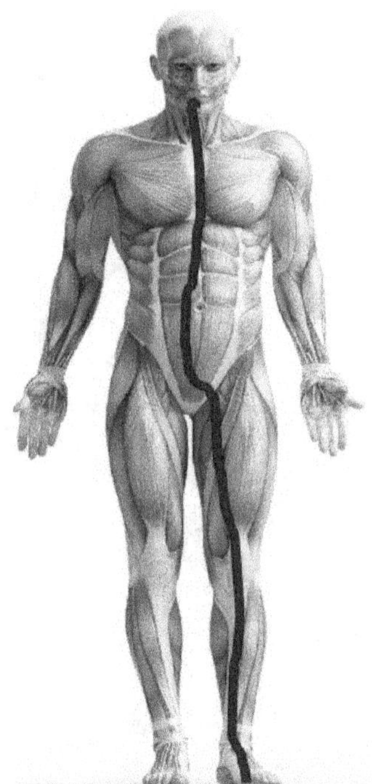

The kidney meridian points run from sole of the foot to muscular bone behind the inner ankle then it goes inner side of legs to top of the thigh and then crosses to spine and enters the kidney, urinary bladder internal to liver, diaphragm and lung and continues to throat and tongue. The main points also run inner thigh to abdomen and the chest to the collar bone.

These points, if exercised properly, will solve - nutrition problems, inside of the legs, sex organs, menstruation, giddiness and kidney troubles.

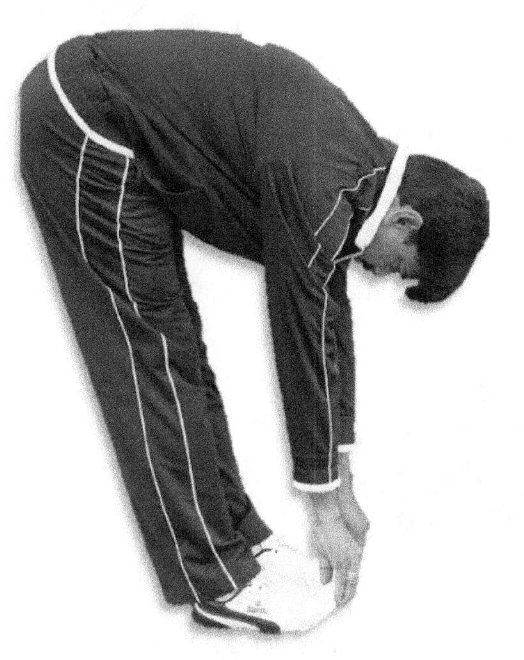

Stand and bend forward and touch the ground and pull the toes up. See Pic1.

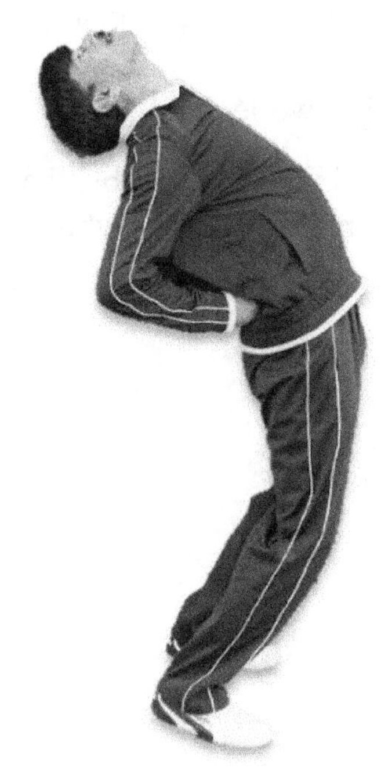

Pic1

Pic2

Stand and bend backwards. See Pic2.

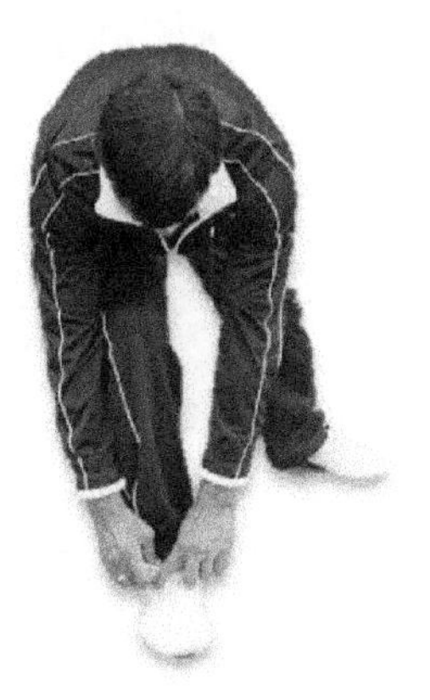

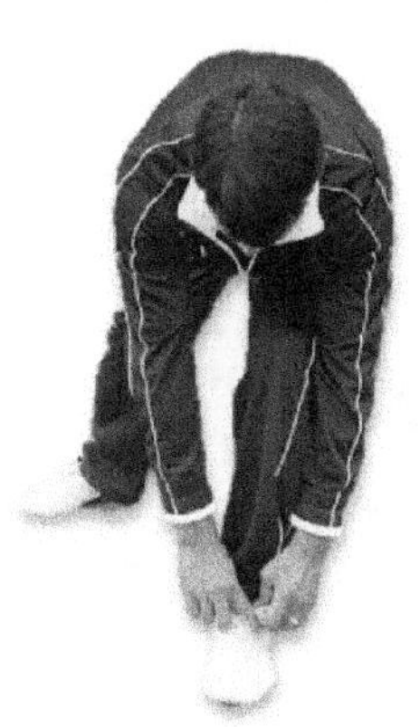

Stand right leg forward and bend as if you are tying shoelace. Do the right leg and left leg and keep doing it for 10 times. This exercise is very good for kidneys.
See the pictures Pic3 and Pic4

Sit with two legs extended and breath in and out. This should be done 25 times daily.

Speread your legs double the shoulder width with hands rest on the ground. Breath in and take hands pull inside legs while breathing in. Come up and bend back then breathout.

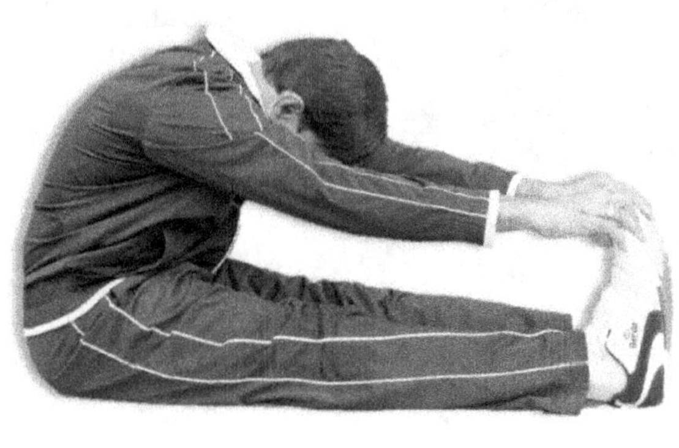

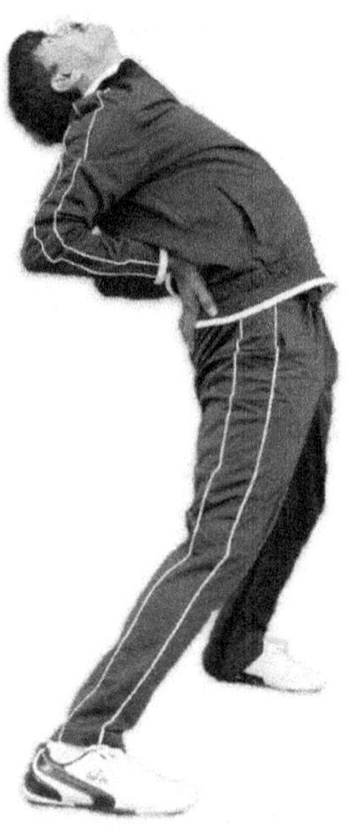

Sit on the chair interlocking the hands and look at the sky and give sound Wooooooo as shown in picture 1

Kidney Sound is WOOOOOOOO and the nature of Kidney color is Black.
Ideal time for doing the healing sound for kidney is between – 5pm to 7pm and the season for Kidneys is winter. One should do this healing sound in front of cedar tree. If you couldn't find a cedar tree, its advisable to do this under any tree that gives pure oxygen.

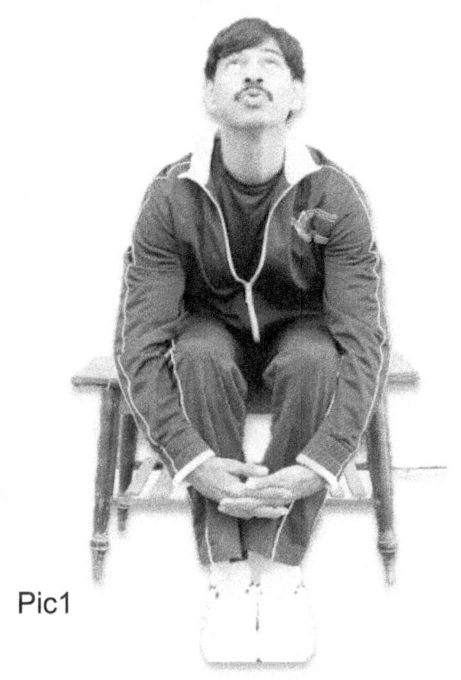

Pic1

Watch Educational films / Read about science articles for healthy kidneys

Liver

Key Functions of Liver

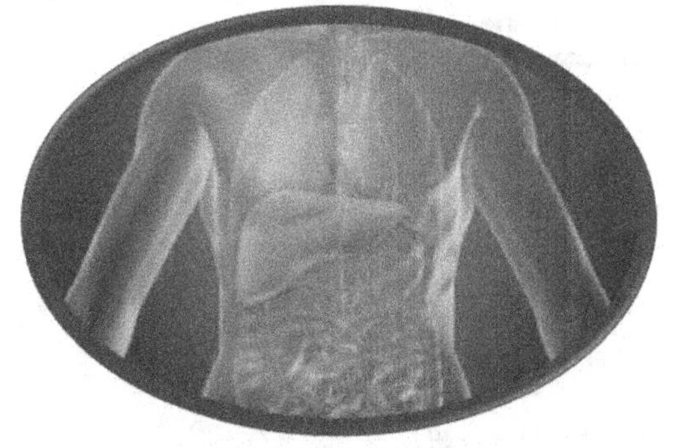

The liver filters and processes blood as it circulates through the body.

It metabolizes nutrients, detoxifies harmful substances, makes blood clotting proteins, and performs many other vital functions.

The cells in the liver contain proteins called enzymes that drive these chemical reactions.

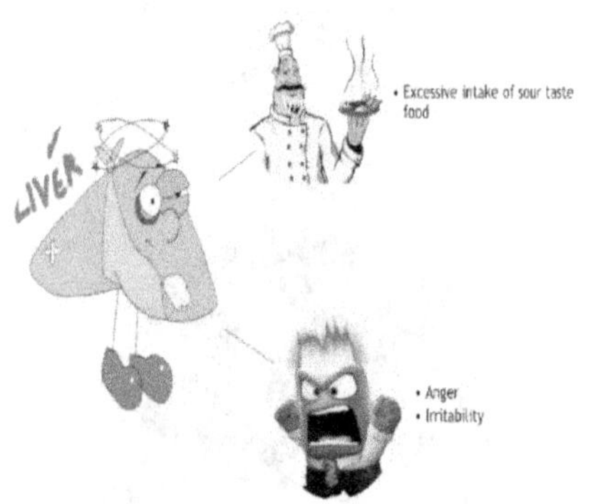

Excess intake of sour taste food will have a negative impact on liver. Also, emotions like anger and irritability will take a toll on Liver.

For Healthy Liver

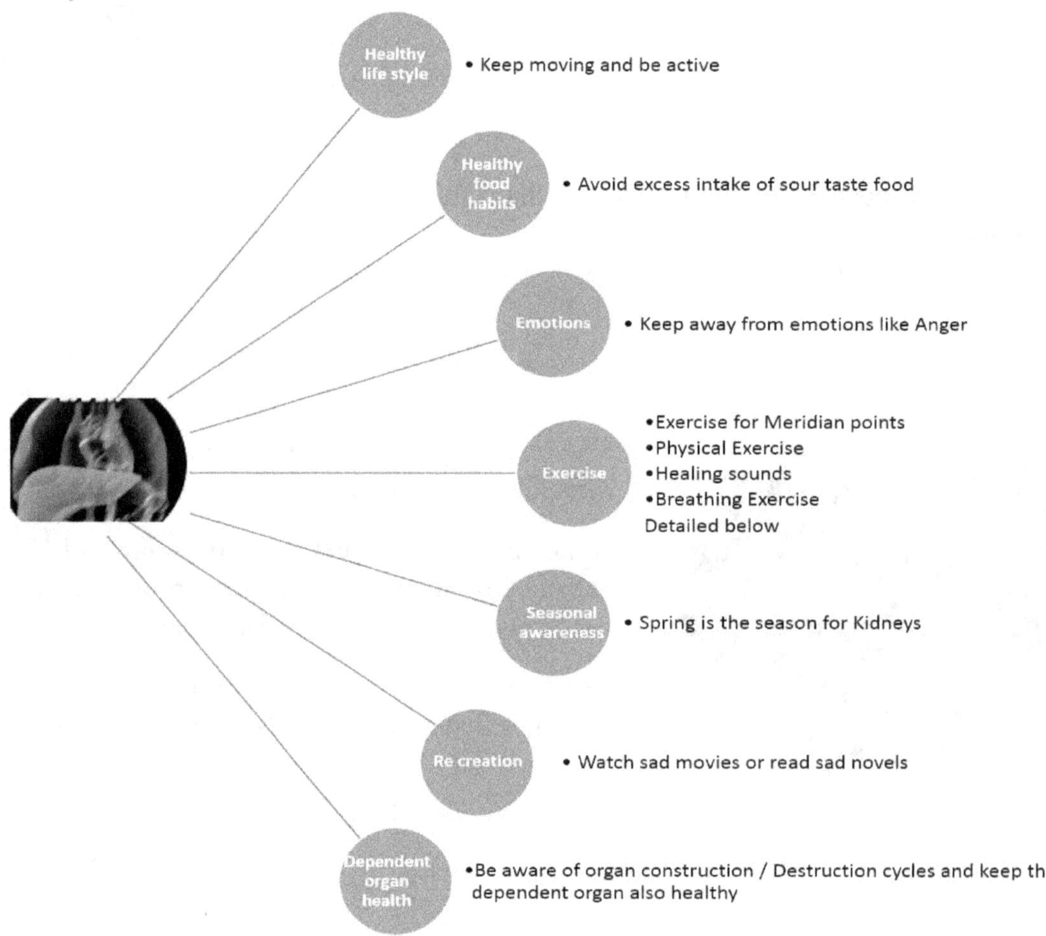

If a person is diagnosed with any type of liver problems, the precautions to be taken are

- ☐ Must avoid excess intake of Sour taste food.
- ☐ Must keep away from emotions like anger.
- ☐ Must be more careful during Spring season.
- ☐ Advisable to watch sad movies or read sad novels.
- ☐ Must take care of associated organ in construction/destruction cycle.
- ☐ Must get engaged in all types of exercises (Physical, breathing, healing sounds and breathing) mentioned.

Exercise for Liver
Physical Exercise for Liver

Massage the navel for at least 1 minute daily in the morning
with left palm for men and right palm for women.
Doing these 20 times will be very beneficial
See Pic 1

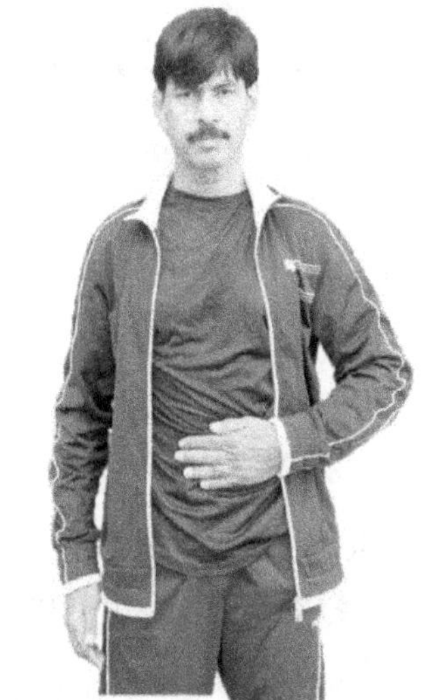

Meridian Points for Liver

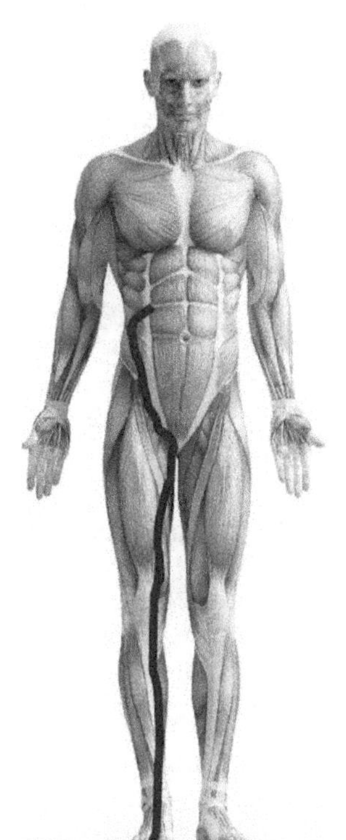

Liver meridian points runs from top
of the big toe and runs upwards
along the back of the foot to inside ankle and goes up inside of the leg
to genital organs and connects to abdomen and goes to rib cage and
connects internally to liver, gall bladder and to lungs goes to throat,
eyes and head

These points must be exercised to get rid of problems related -
digestion, chest, inside of legs and liver

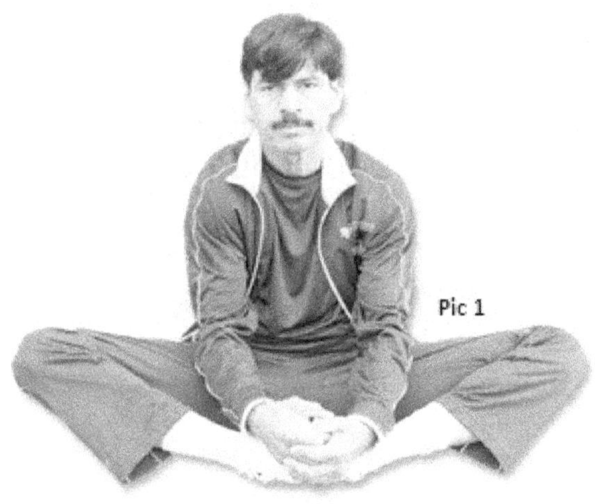

Pic 1

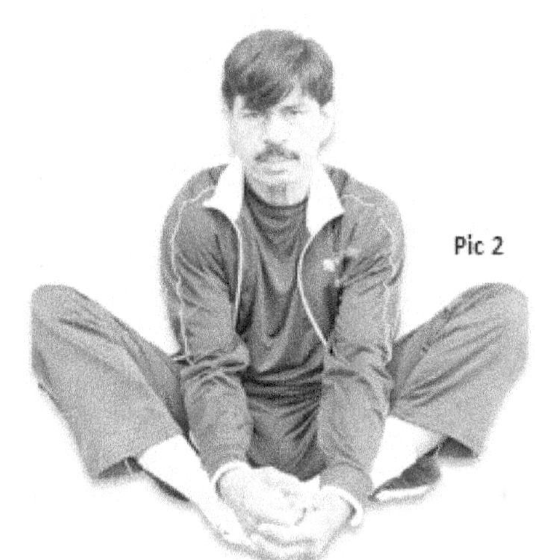

Pic 2

Sit-down and touch left sole and right sole and hold feed with your hands and shake thighs.

This good for liver and inner side of legs. Do this for 30 secs to 1 minute daily.

Sit on one leg and other leg extended without bending. Do this exercise for 10 times each. Note: You must sit, get up and sit on another leg.

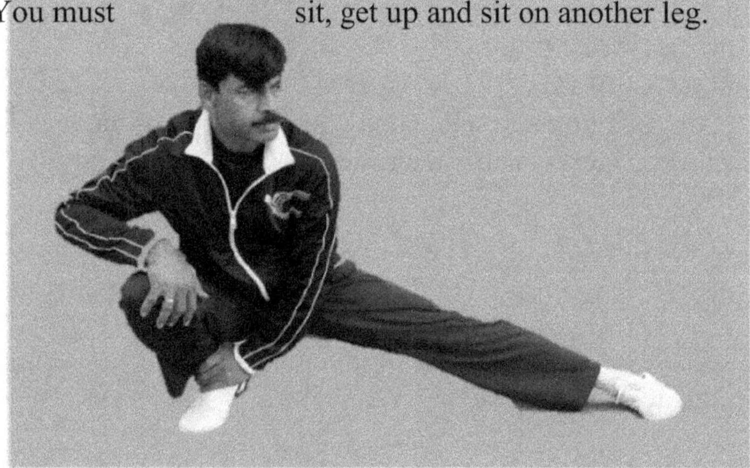

Variation: Lie down with knees bent, and split the bent knees and shake legs like a butterfly as shown in the pictures 1 and 2 below..

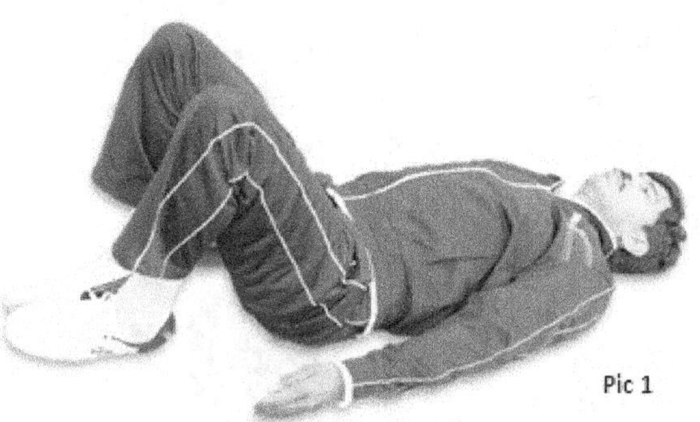

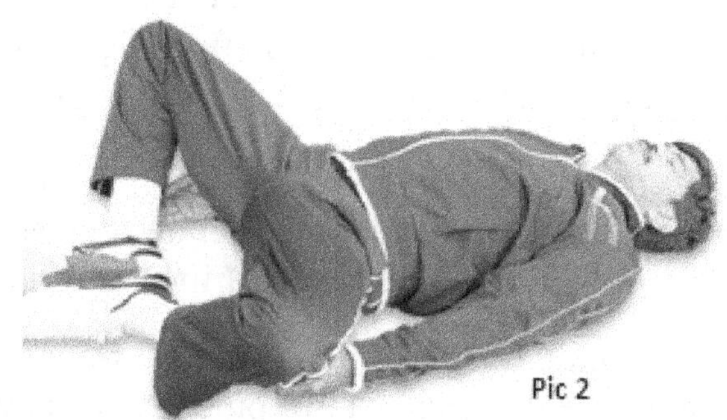

Stand on one leg and lift the other leg straight
up towards the side as shown in the pictures below. Try to reach from Pic1 picture to Pic3.

Doing these 20 times will be very
beneficial for
liver.

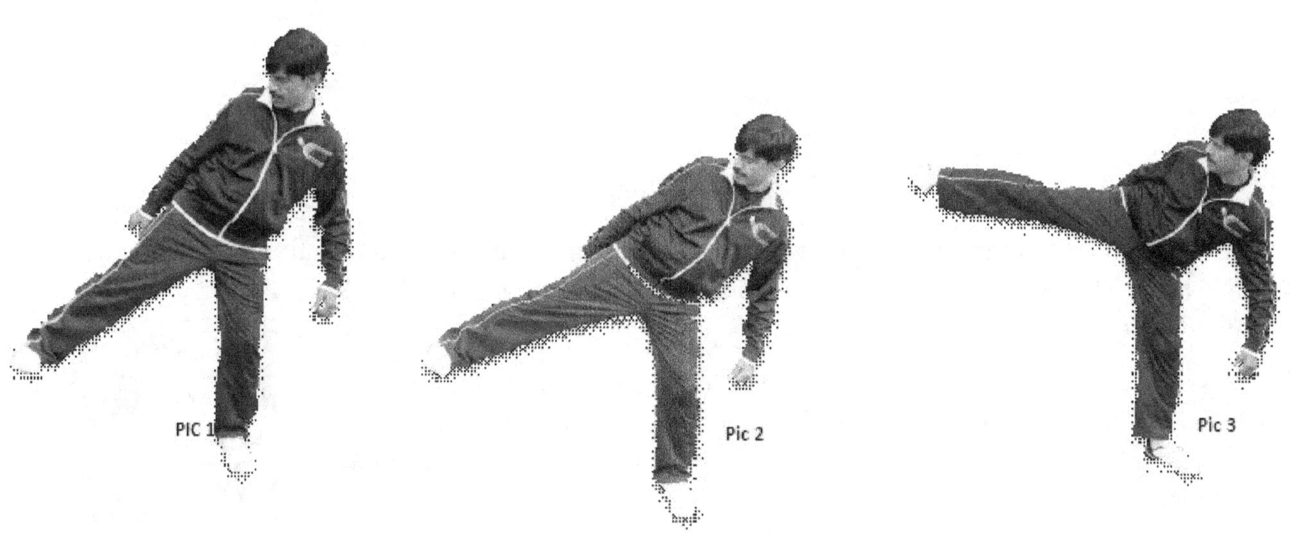

Healing sounds for Liver

Sit on chair or table and interlock the fingers and raise your hands over the head and turn slightly to the left so that right ribs and chest contract. Please see the picture.

Liver Sound is SHSHSHSHSHSH and the nature of Liver color is Green. Ideal time for doing healing sounds for liver is between – 1am to 3am and the season for liver is spring.

One should do this healing sound in front of pineapple tree (pine tree). If you couldn't find a pine tree, its advisable to do this under any tree that gives pure oxygen.

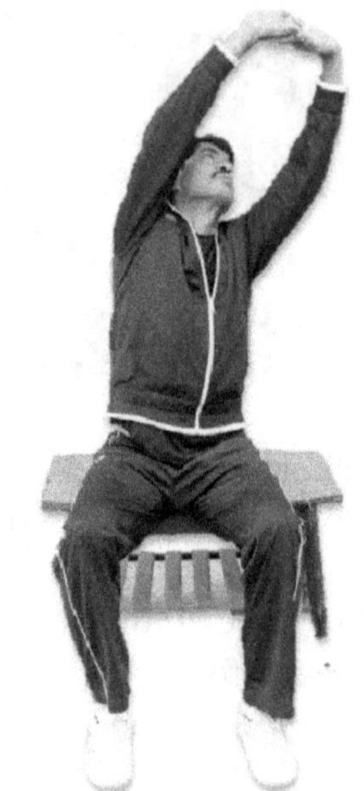

Other tips for healthy liver

One must read sad novels or watch sad movies for healthy liver

Stomach.

Key functions of Stomach

The stomach can expand to temporarily store food. Partial digestion of the food takes place here. The churning action of the stomach muscles physically breaks down the food.

The stomach releases acids and enzymes for the chemical breakdown of food. The enzyme pepsin is responsible for protein breakdown. The stomach releases food into the small intestine in a controlled and regulated manner.

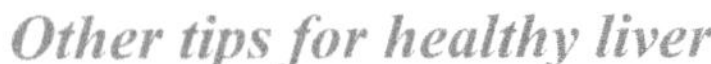

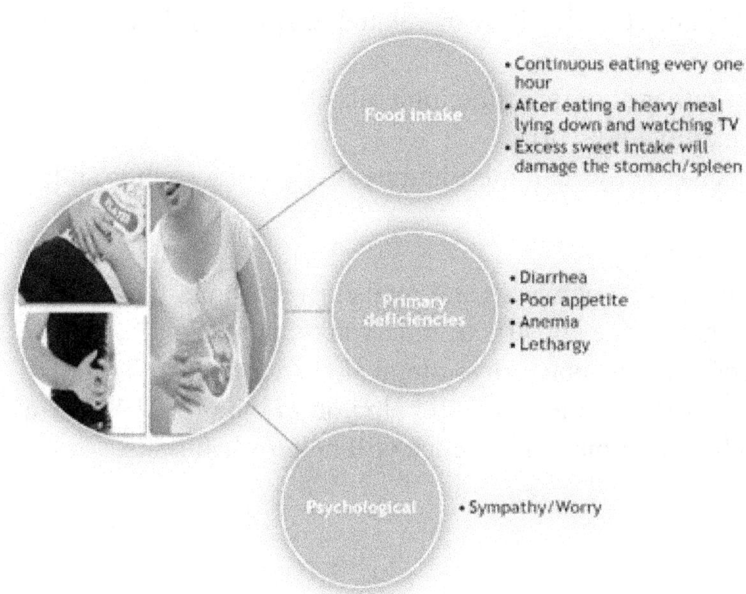

The food we eat,
inherent stomach deficiencies
and emotions will play a crucial
role in deteriorating
the stomach's health.

For healthy stomach

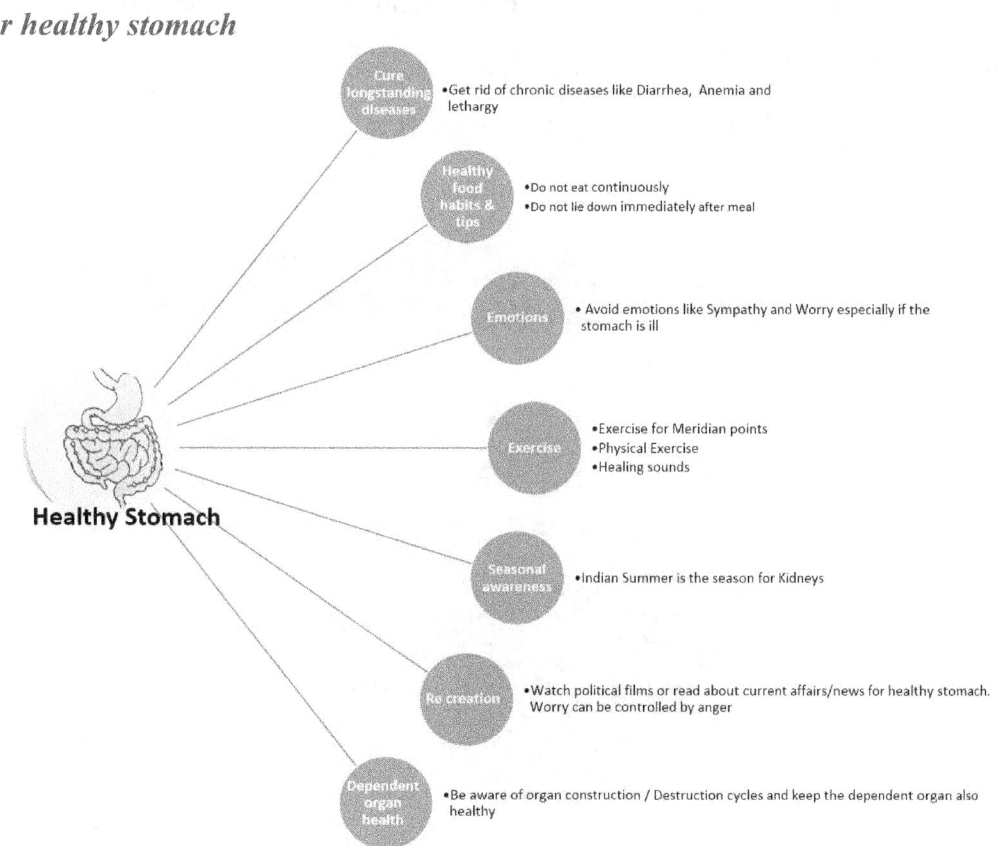

If a person is diagnosed with any stomach related ailment, the person:

- Must take extra caution to get rid of chronic ailments related to stomach (like Anemia/lethargy)
- Must not eat continuously, but rather at define time intervals
- Must avoid emotions like Sympathy and worry.
- Must do the organ related exercises (Physical, meridian points, healing sounds and breathing)
- Must be more careful during summer
- Advisable to watch political films/documentaries and read current affairs
- Must take care of associated organ in the construction/destruction cycle.
- Avoid extreme over eating food – it has many physiological, psychological including metabolic causes. There is no medical or therapy will help you in long run. It's like a putting a poison in the stomach and no medical science will help re-habilitate.

Exercise for Stomach

The below said physical exercise will keep the stomach Meridian Points for Stomach.

The below said physical exercise will keep the stomach healthy.

Lie down and then touch your thighs to chest. Repeat this for 10mins a day.

See the pictures 1 and 2.

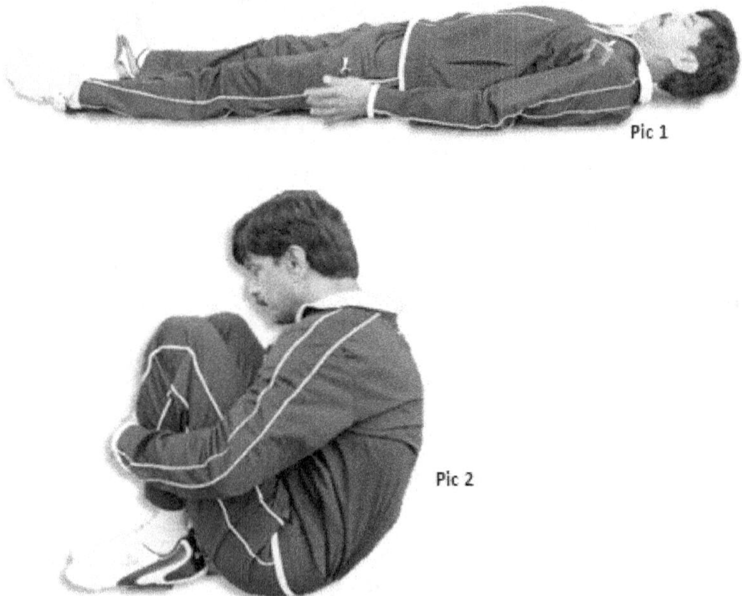

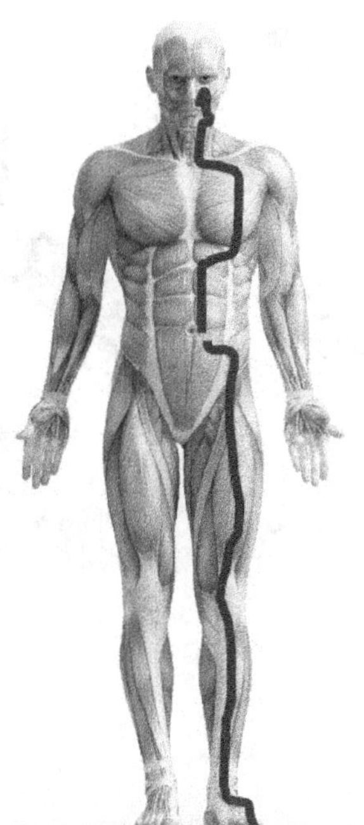

The stomach meridian points begin at the side of the nose and runs to the inner corner of the eyes below the eyeball and then descends to upper gums and curve around the lips then goes to the lower jaws and then passes upwards to the front of the ear near the fore head. From jaws it also runs down along the throat above the collarbone, enters the stomach and connect to spleen internally.

The other points run from middle toe to knee and thigs and joins to the spleen meridian.

If these points are properly exercised, we can get rid of diseases related to - stomach, intestinal, eyes, nose, mouth, ears, and chest and outside legs

Stomach Meridian Exercise

Lie down and spread legs and get up and touch the left toe and right toe alternating. Doing these 10 times will be very beneficial for stomach. See the pictures 1, 2 and 3

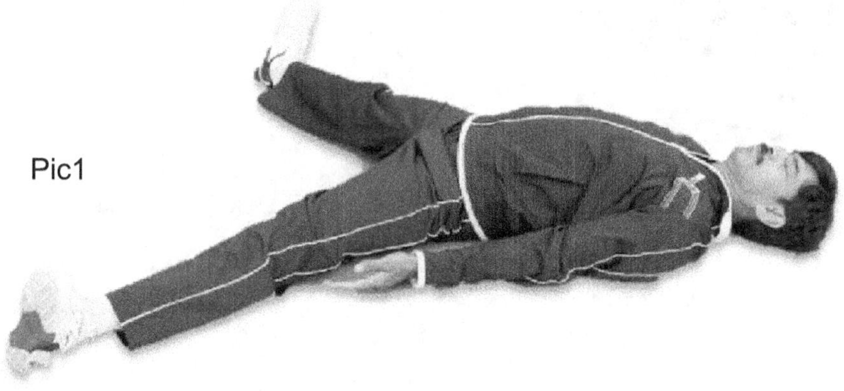

Pic1

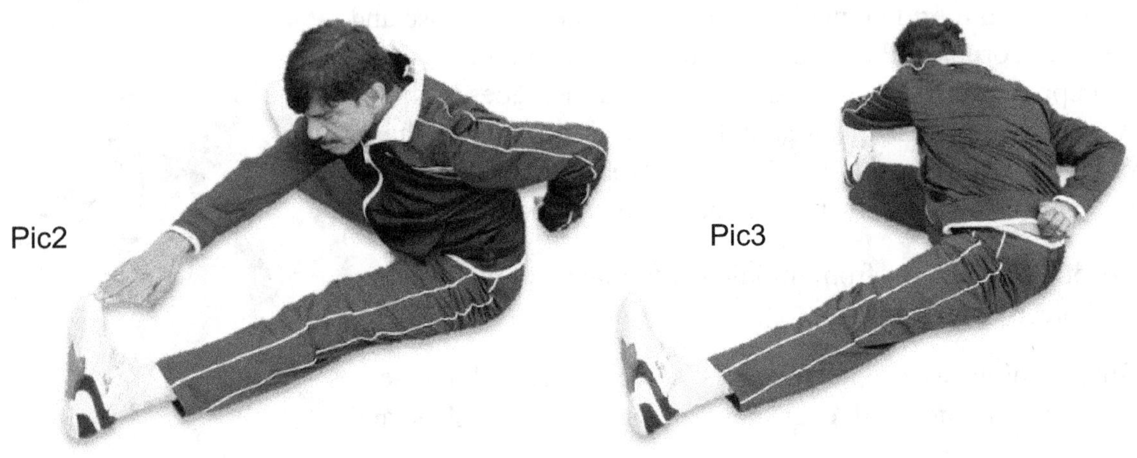

Pic2   Pic3

This exercise is to be done by locking your foot to a wall or step and press your upper body and keep the spinal cord straight and then inhale and exhale while holding the legs. Repeat 10 times

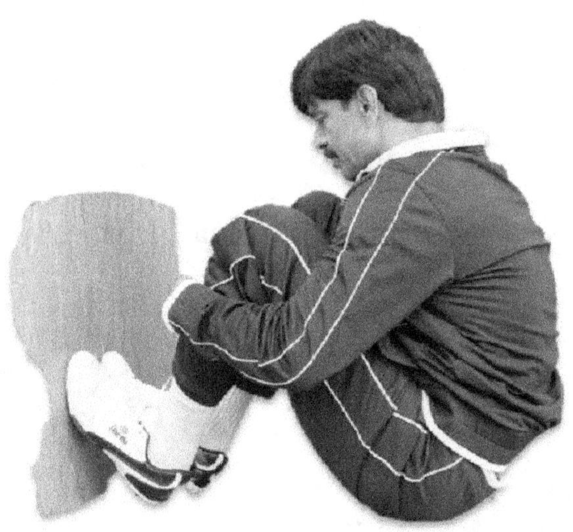

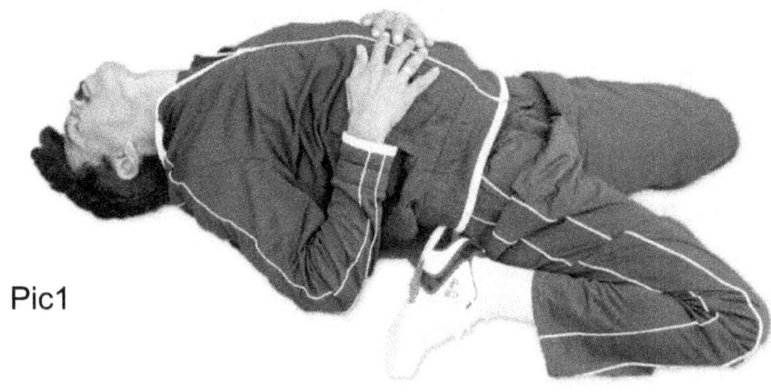

Pic1

Bend your two legs at knee outside the body and lie down. This exercise is very good for stomach as all the meridian points are connected to organs.

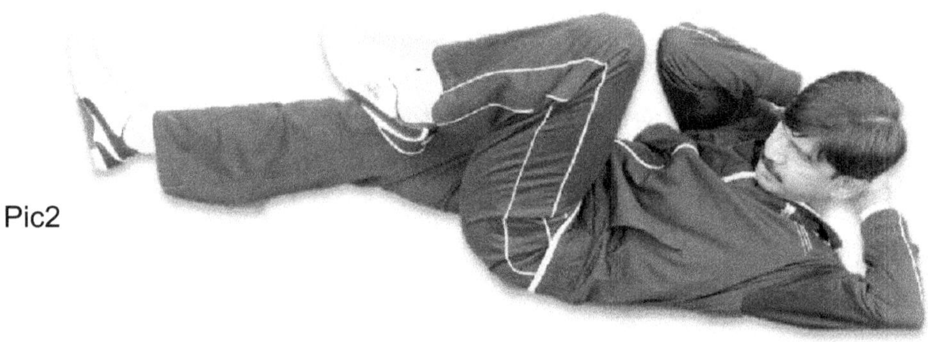

Pic2

In this exercise, you must peddle the legs with elbow touching the knees every time you do alternatively. Doing these 20 times each side will be very beneficial for abdominal health. See Pic2 and Pic3

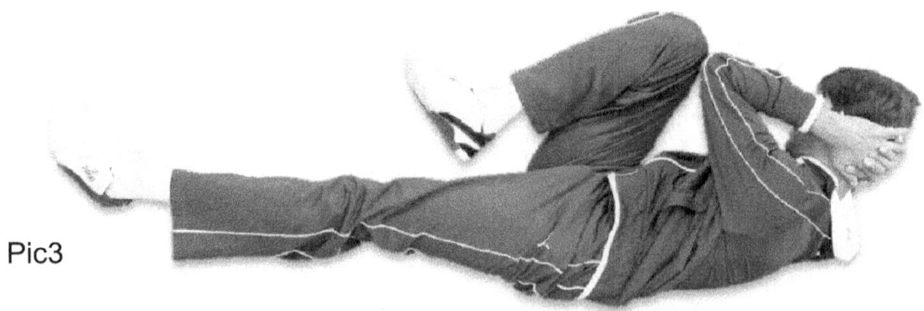

Pic3

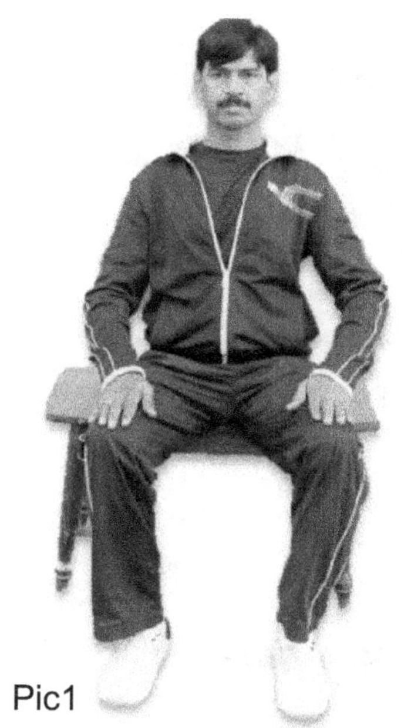

Pic1

Sit on the chair with hands on the lap and and press finger tips to the solar plex and do the stomach sound VUUU…Then come back to hands on the lap after each sound. Then feel stomach is Yellow color for 10 seconds. see pictures 1 and 2

Stomach Sound is VUUUUUUU *and the nature* of Stomach color is Yellow.

Ideal time to do the healing sounds for healthy stomach is between - *7AM* to 9AM *and*

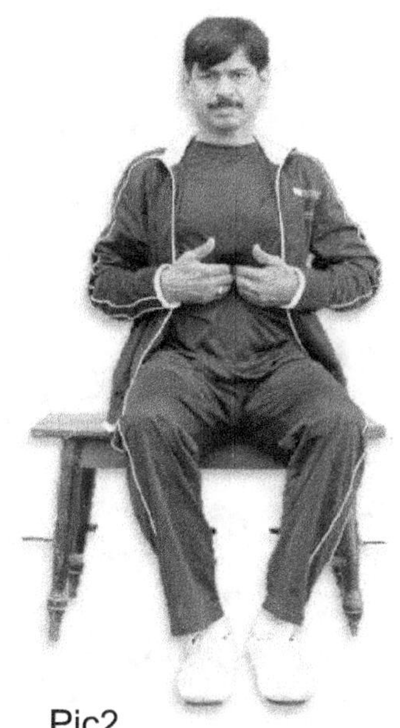

Pic2

*the s*eason for Stomach is Indian *summer*.

Doing this exercise in front of willow tree is good and will get immediate results. If you are not near to willow trees, one should do this near any tree/plant with pure oxygen.

Meridian Points in left palm

Meridian Points in Right palm.

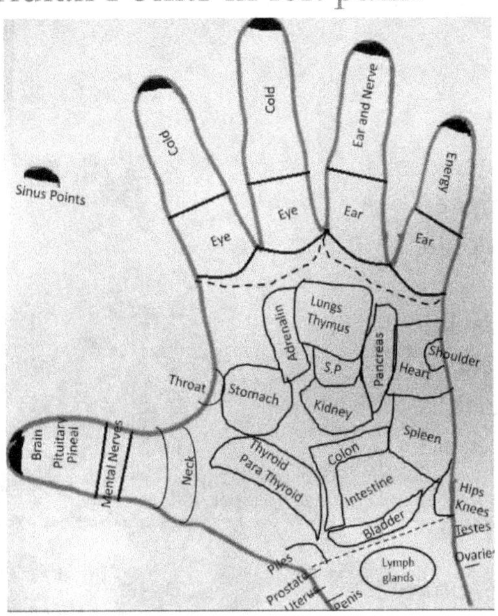

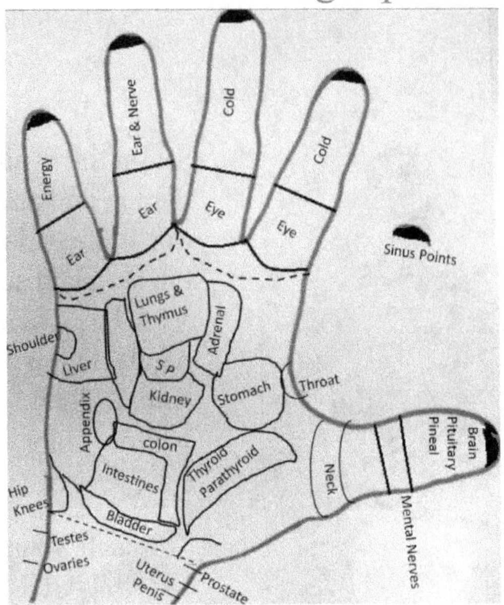

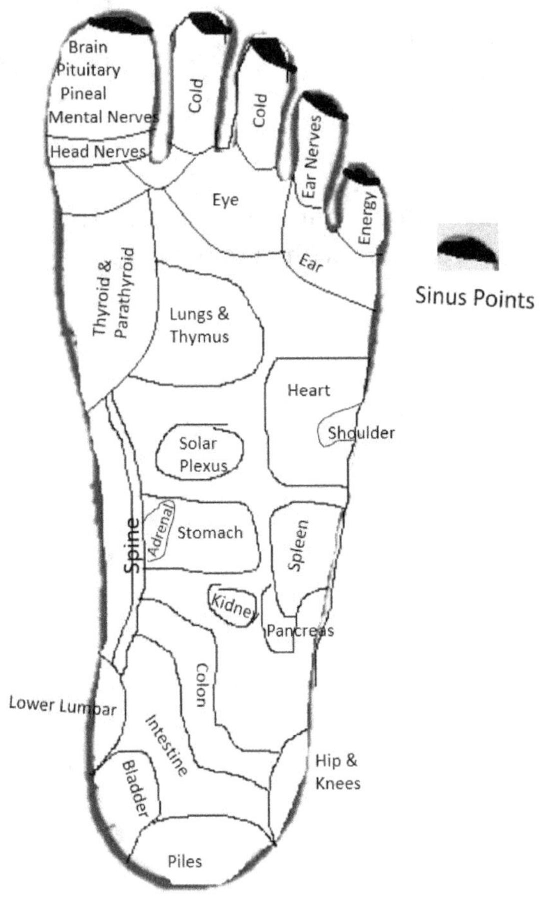

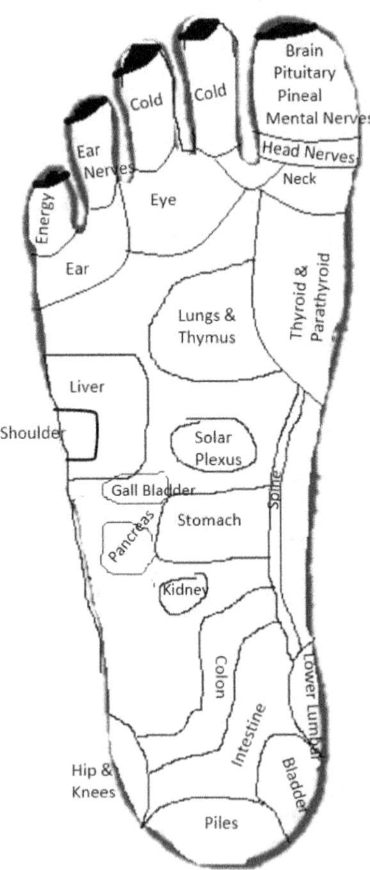

Various categories of exercises for Longevity

a) Golden Eight Secret Health Exercises
b) Diamond martial yoga exercises
c) Medicinal Energy
d) Medicinal Martial Yoga Massage
e) Advanced Medicinal Martial Yoga Exercises

For all the exercises that are detailed below, a note

Breath in with tongue adhered to raft of the mouth and breath out with the lower abdomen. Tongue should be taken out while breathing out.

Golden Eight

8 Bagua (PaKua) internal and external exercises equip one with a healthy and disease free body. These are popularly called as golden Eight or 8 Broacde or 8 Baduanjin or 8 forms in China and other countries. These golden eight are practiced with sitting , standing and moving. These exercises are practiced thousands of years by our ancient monks and Yogis for longevity.

First Golden exercise

Put right palm on the neck and left reverse palm on the lower back and twist back side and opposite side. Put left palm on the neck and left revere palm on the lower back and twist back side of right with breath in while twisting and breathe out while coming back to normal position.

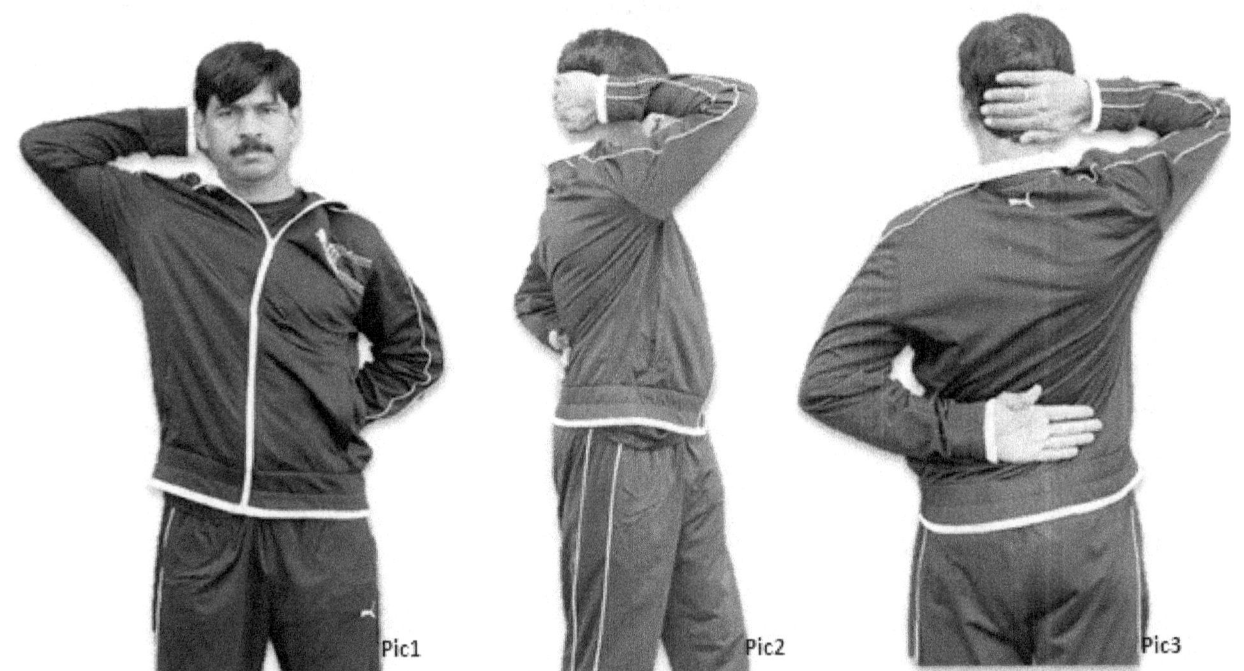

This exercise is advised to be done 6 to 12 times every day.

Second Golden exercise

Horse stance and extend your left hand with twisting upright of the wrist and turn. Breath in while moving to the other direction. Breath out while extending the other hand like bow and arrow hit, strain your arms.

Stand and extend right palm upwards as if you are holding the sky and press the ground with

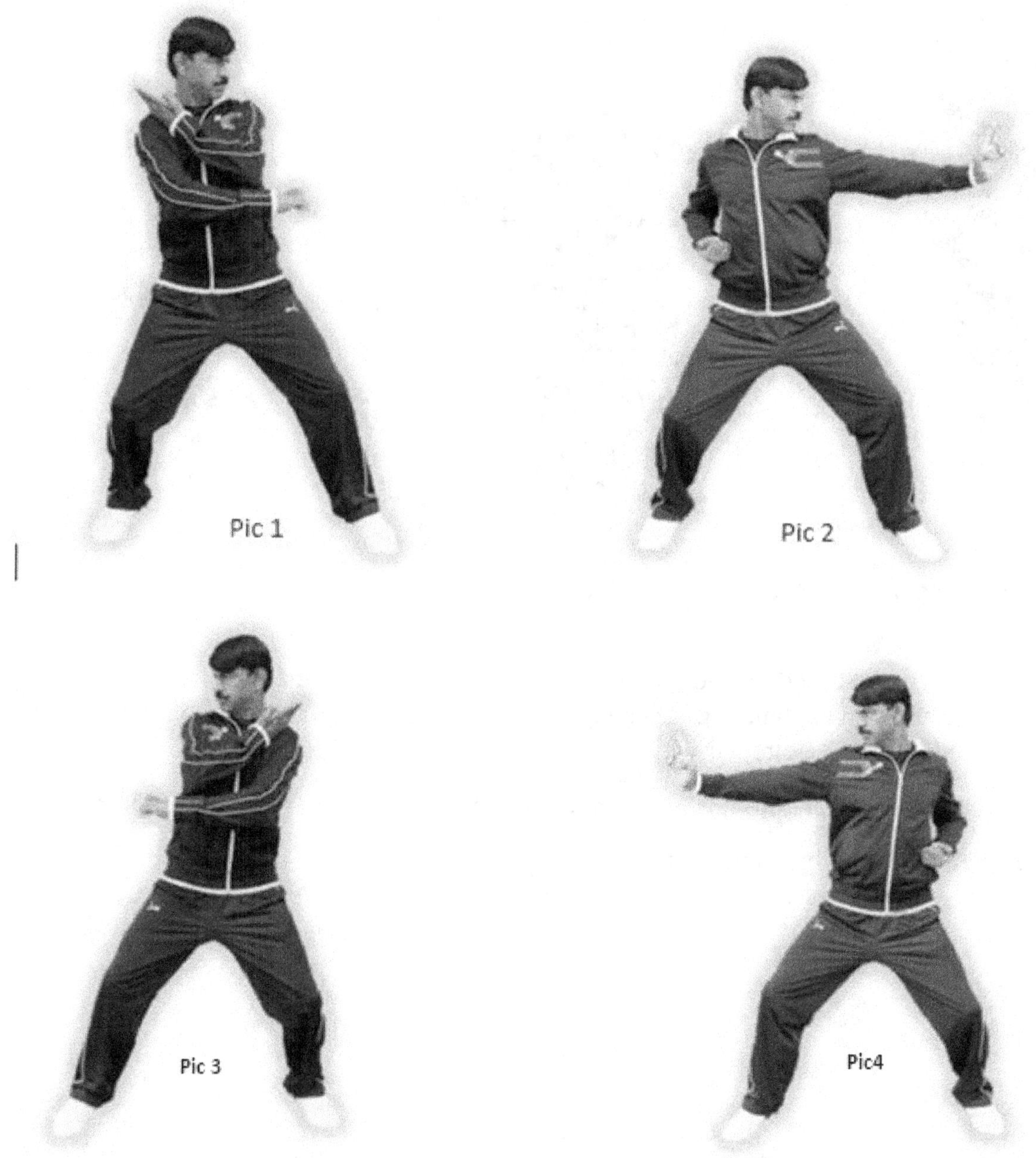

palm. This should be done simultaneously and feel you are pressing the sky and earth at the same time.   Please see the pictures 1, 2 and 3

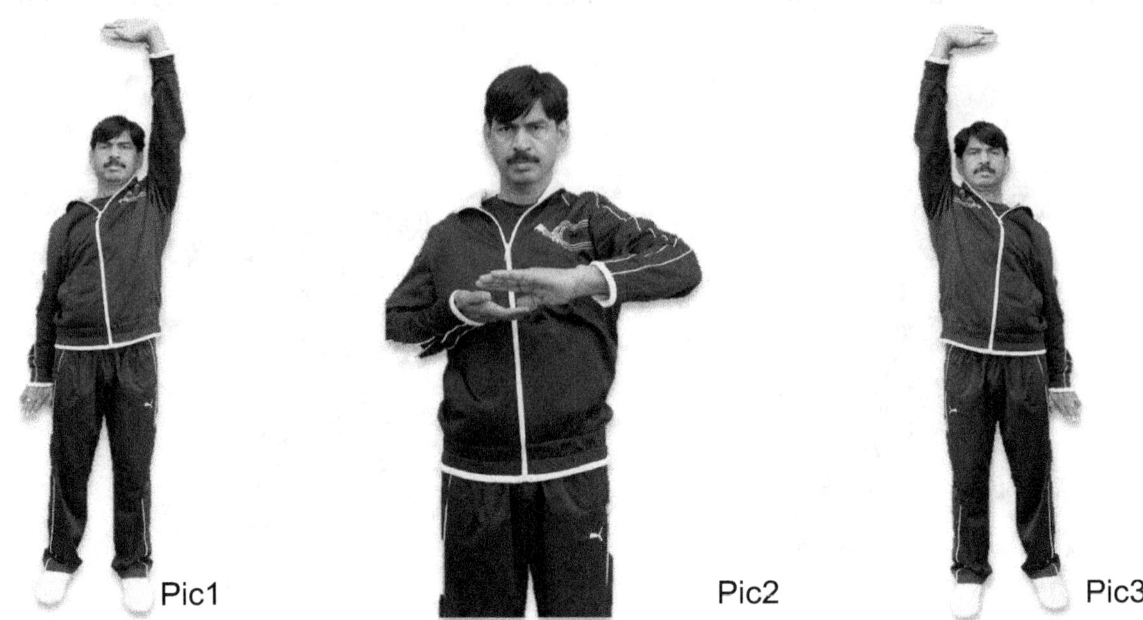

This exercise is advised to be done 6 times every day.

Fourth Golden exercise

Stand and interlock hands and extend maximum with raising hand to the overhad as if you are tied up to a pole and you are hanging. Then slowly bring the hands to the sides and bring back as shown in the picture, in a circular way.

Breath in with tongue adhered to raft of the mouth and breath out with the lower abdomen. Tongue should be taken out while breathing out.

This exercise is advised to be done 6 times every day.

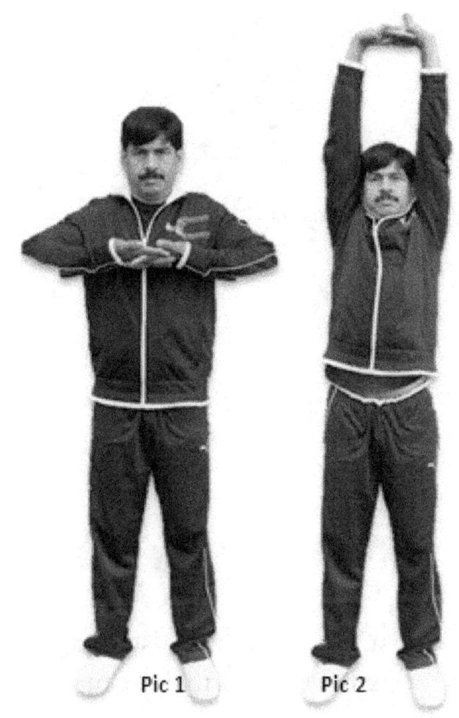

Pic 1   Pic 2

Fifth Golden exercise

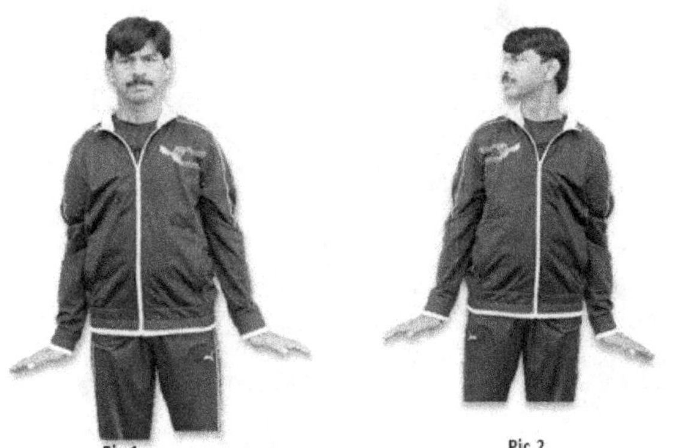

Pic 1   Pic 2

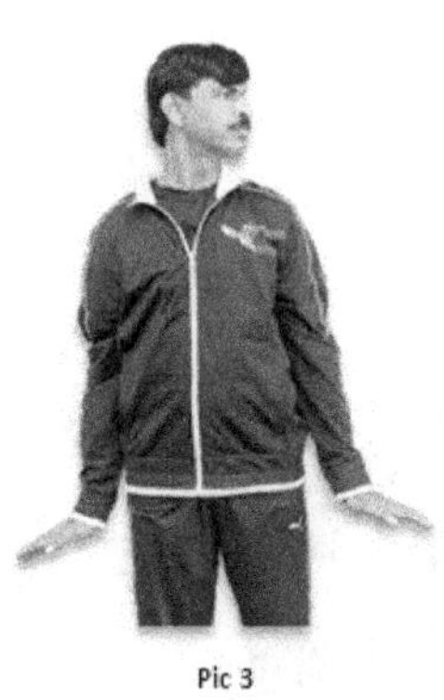

Pic 3

Stand and hands sideways with palm facing ground (bend at the wrist). Breathe in and stretch in and out. Turn left and right side slowly. Please see the pictures 1, 2 and 3 below. This exercise is advised to be done 6 times every day.

Sixth Golden exercise

Horse stance and punch left slowly with breath in ; turn to other direction and punch out the other hand with breath out.

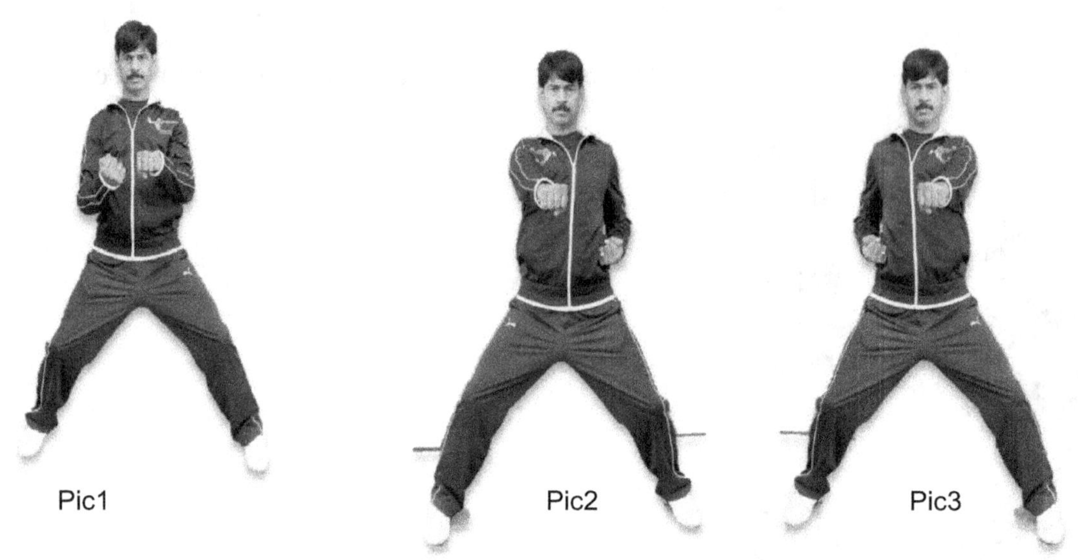

<table>
<tr><td>Pic1</td><td>Pic2</td><td>Pic3</td></tr>
</table>

This exercise is advised to be done 6 times every day.

Seventh Golden exercise

Standing in Horse stance, put your hands on the knees and twist to the left and also to right. Breath in while twisting to the side and breath out while coming back to normal position. This exercise is advised to be done 6 times every day.

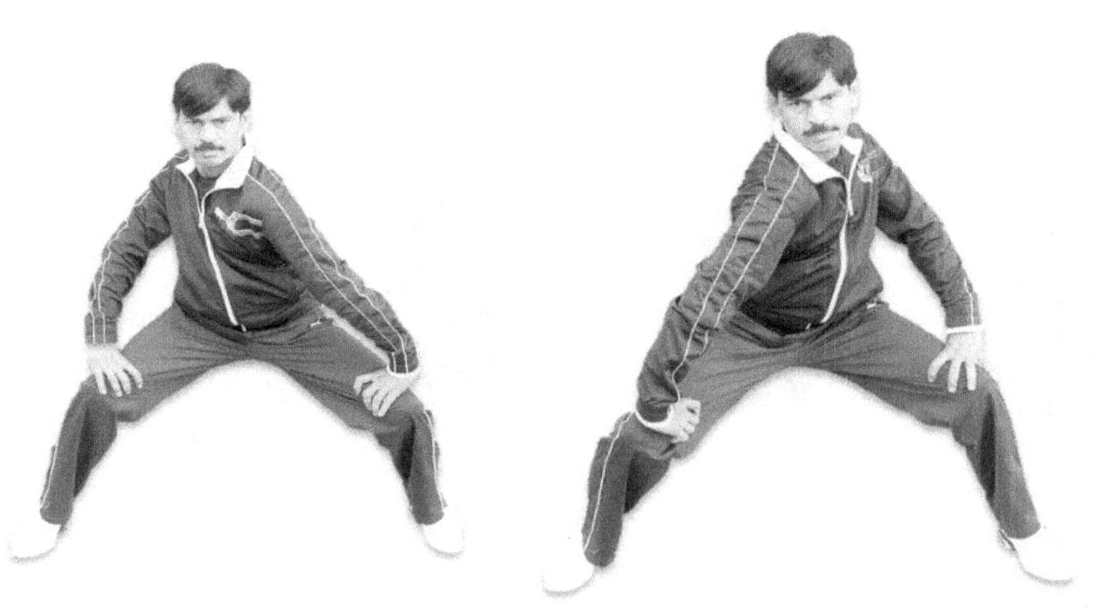

Stand and put your palms on the lower back and bend backwards maximum with breath in; bend forwards with breath out. These exercises are advised to be done 6 times every day.

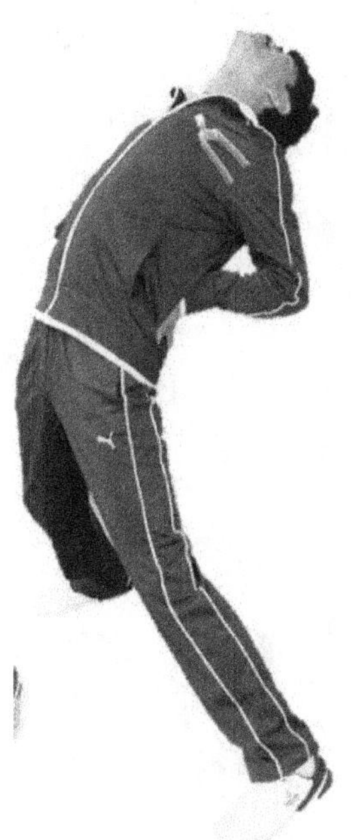

Diamond Nine Exercises

Diamond Exercise I Stand and run on the spot at least 10 seconds.

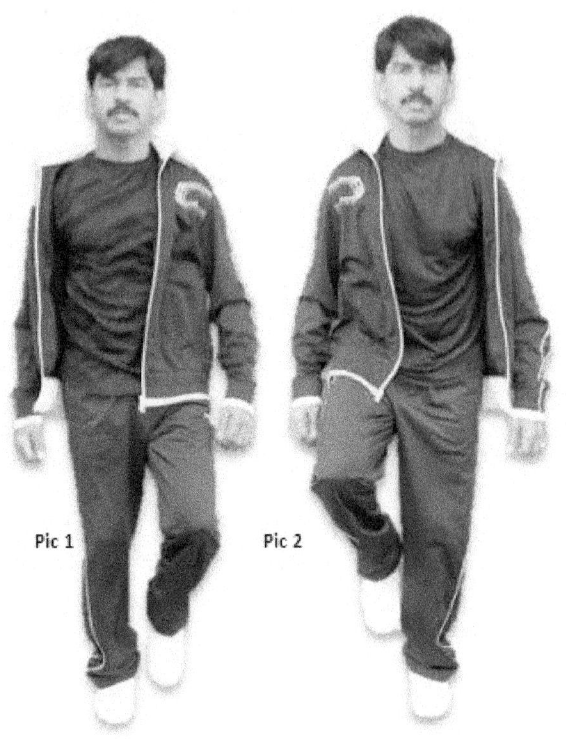

Diamond Exercise II Lie down with hands on the hips and raise your hips and legs

Do cycling at least 5 times

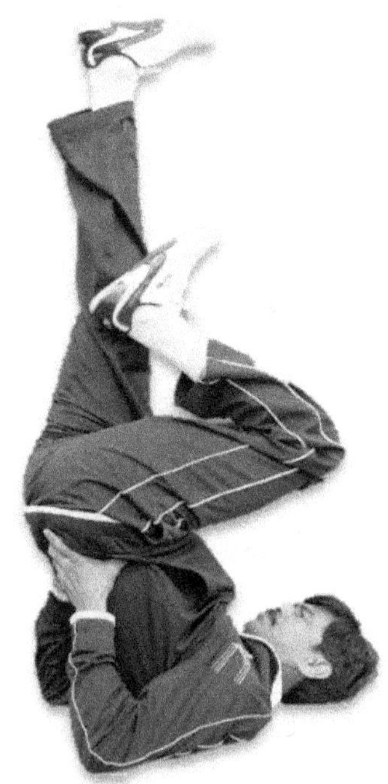

Diamond Exercise III **Keep your hands beyond your back Hit the ground with your legs at least 6 to 12 times**

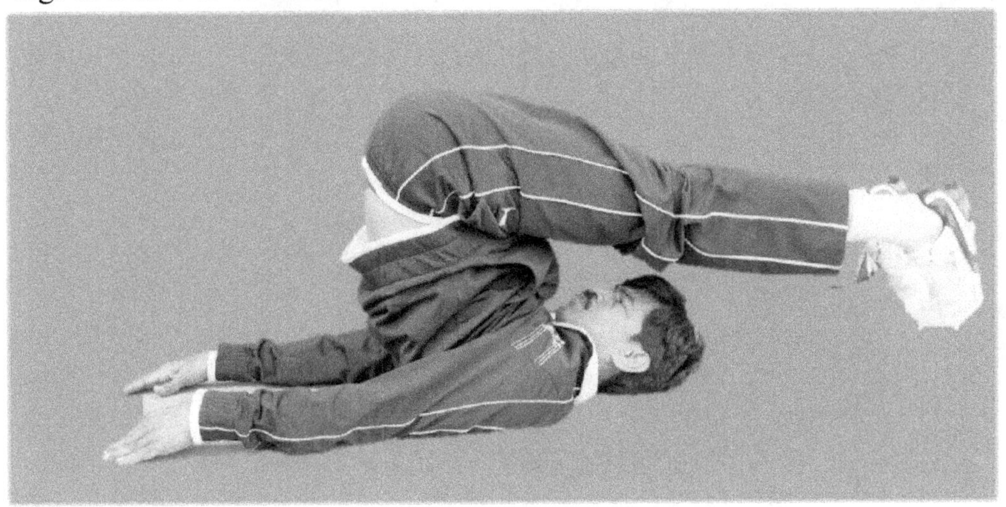

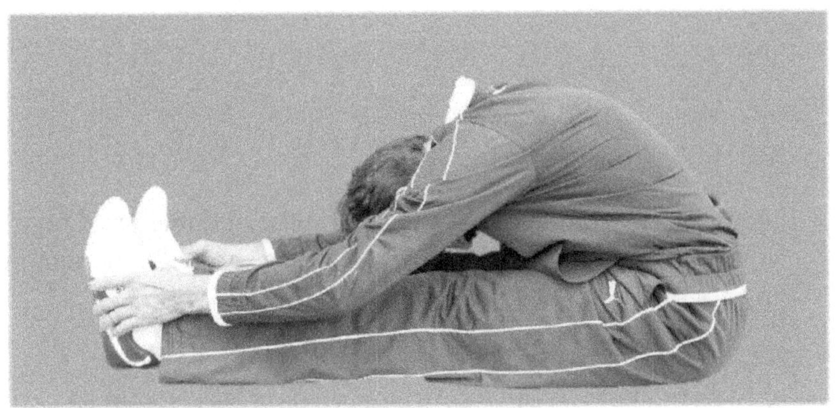

Diamond Exercise IV Bend forward. Touch your head to the knees.
Do it for 2 times

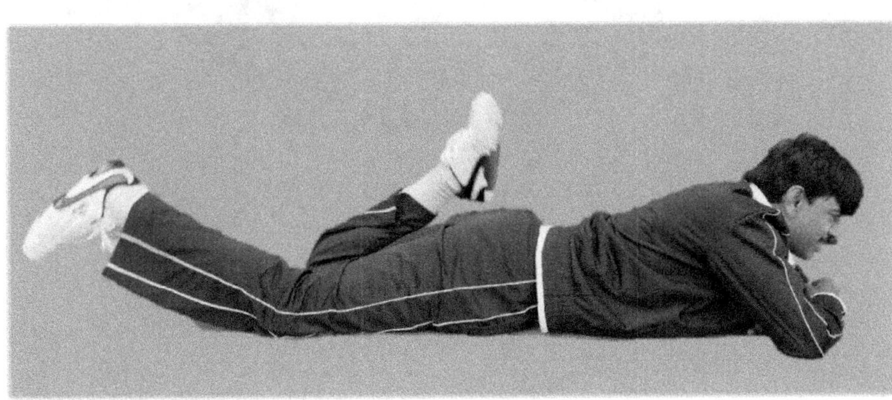

Diamond Exercise V
Lie down as shown in the picture.

Hit your buttocks with the ball of the foot for 2 times

Diamond Exercise VI Hold your ankle and lift your upper body and legs to the maximum

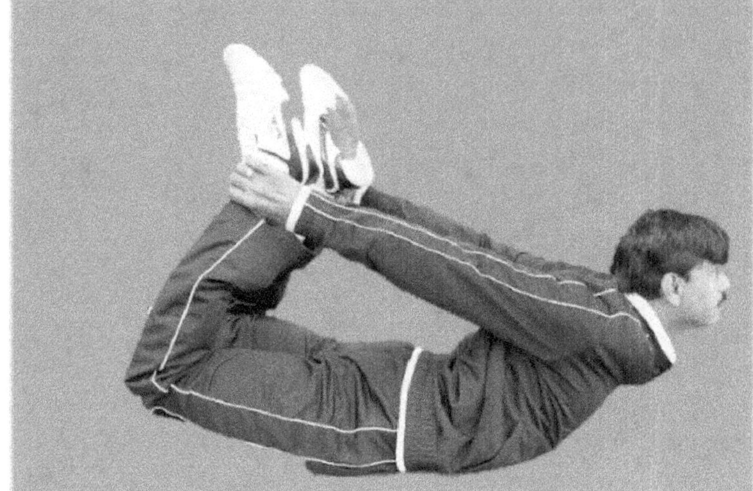

Diamond Exercise VII Kneel and stretch your tongue out maximum with eyes wide open

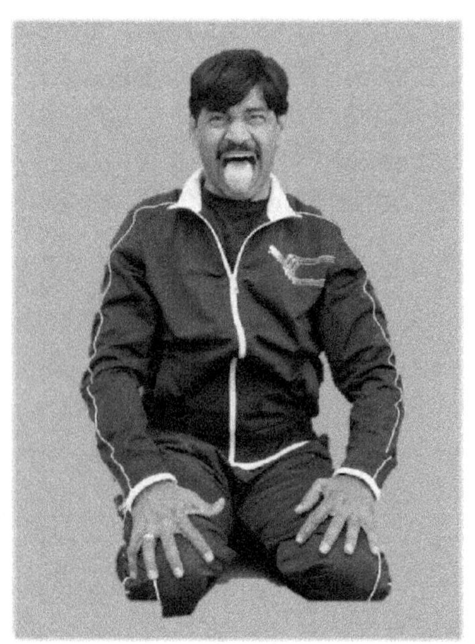

Diamond Exercise VIII – Lie down on the abdomen and raise your legs and hands to the maximum as shown in the picture.

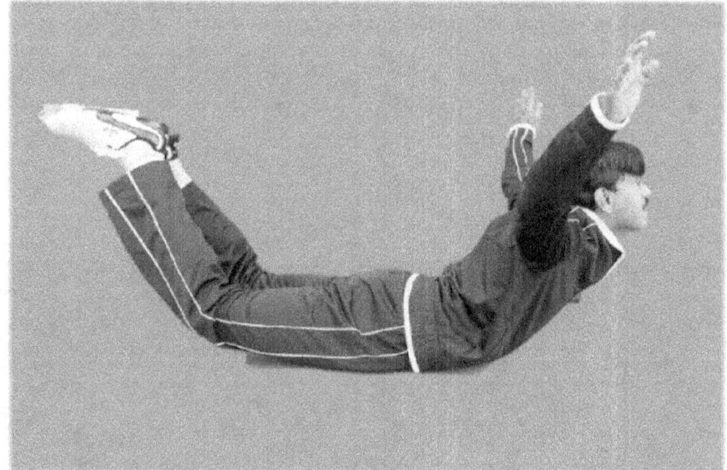

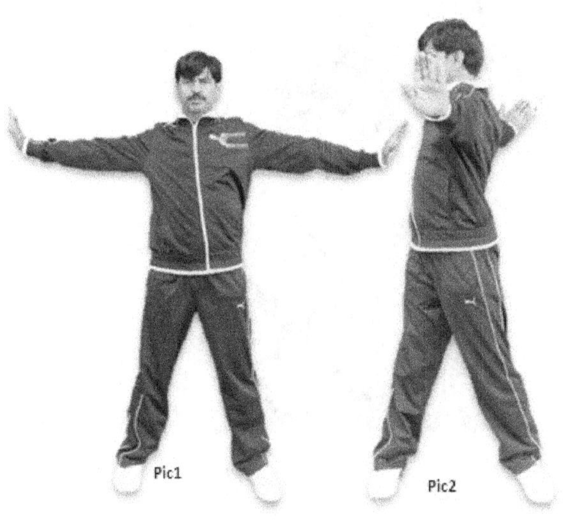
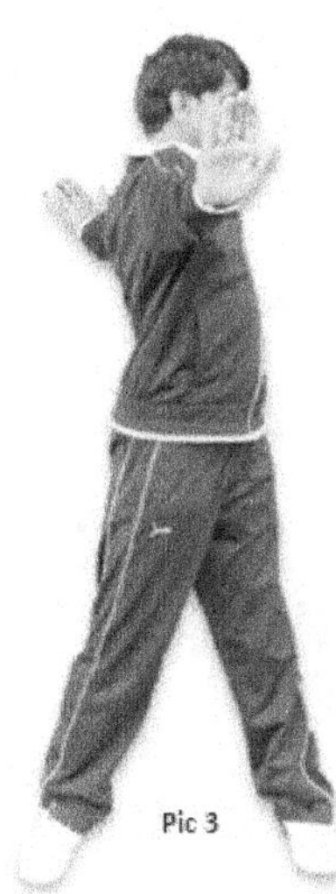

Diamond IX Horse stance and spread hands sideways without bending elbows and twist upper body. See the pictures Pic1 through Pic3

Medicinal Massage Exercises

AI Sit with legs crossed as shown in the picture. Rub hands till hod and message total face including ear. Similarly massage right shoulder and left shoulder. This should be done 6 times clockwise and 6 times anticlockwise.

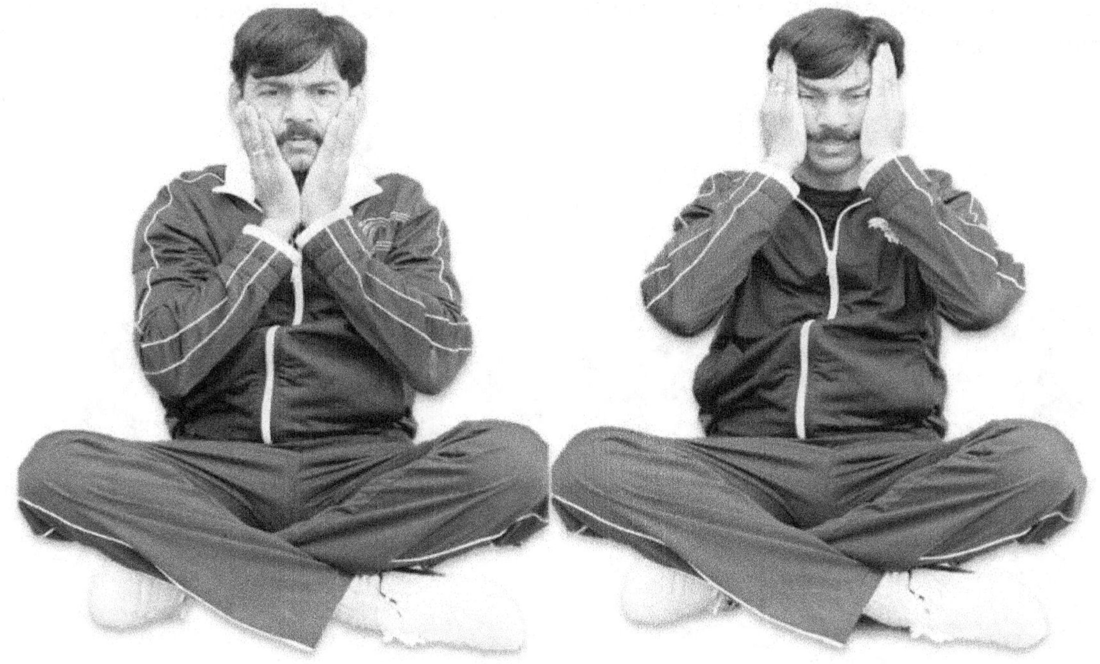

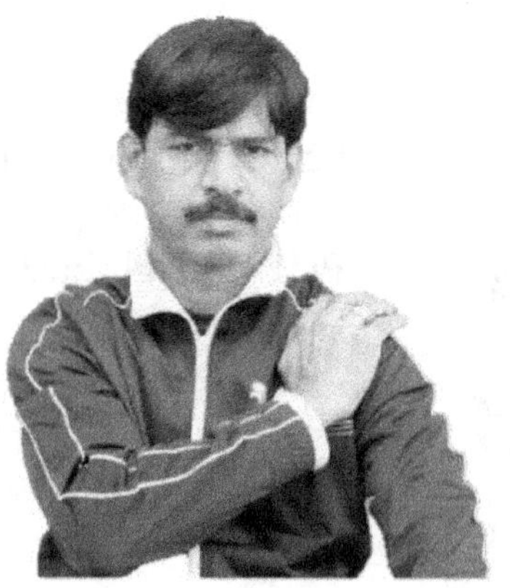 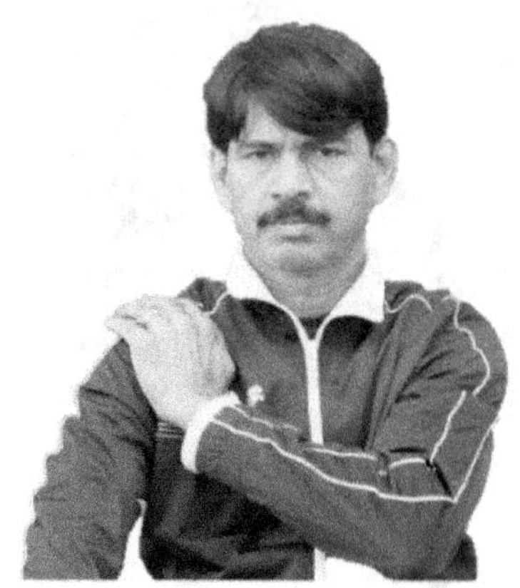

AII Massage the shoulder symmetrically
clockwise and anti-clockwise. It is advisable to do this 12 times per day.

AIII Massage the knees symmetrically clockwise and anticlockwise. It is advisable to
do this 12 times per day.

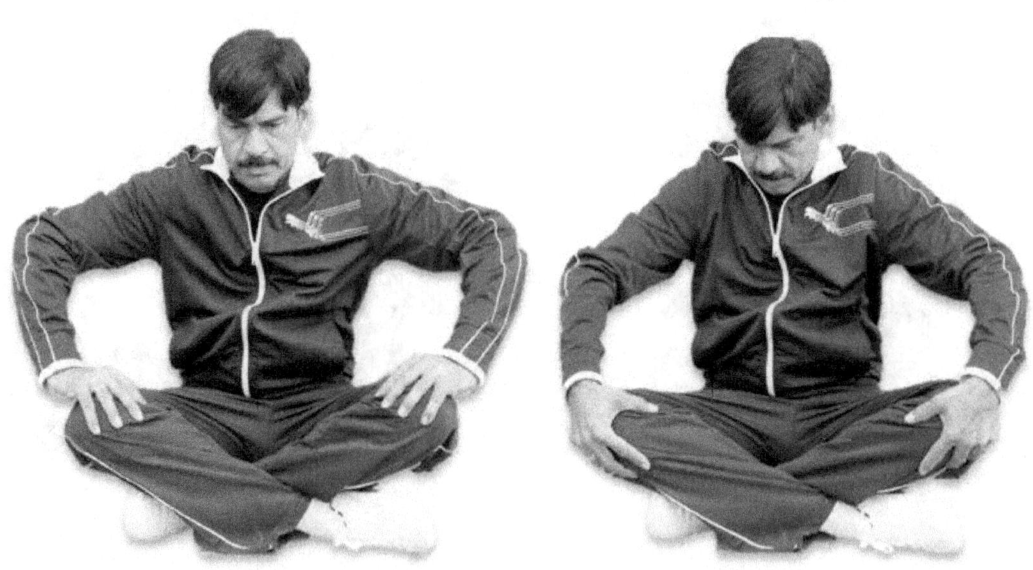

AIV Massage side of nose with index fingers; rub the index finger with palm by warming and massage the nose corner 36 times. Refer the pictures below

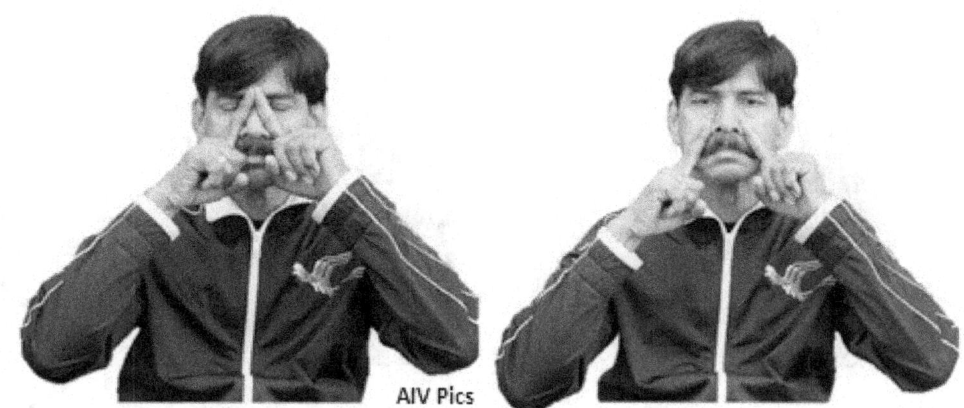

AIV Pics

AV Massage the ears 20 secs with two hands.

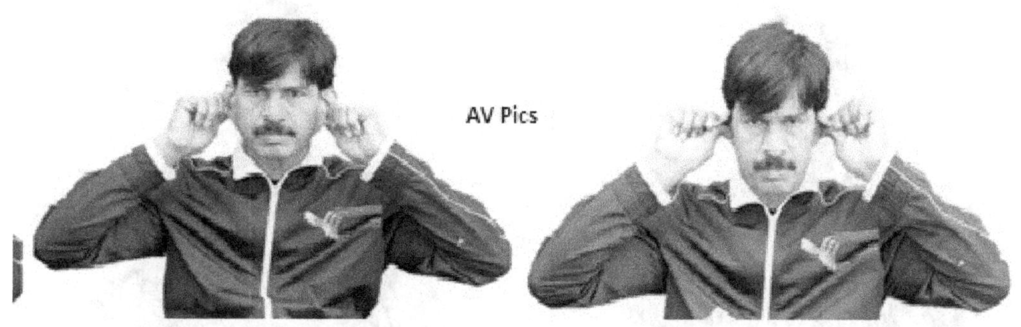

AV Pics

AVI Massage the palms and massage the back for half minute.
And also. hit with your wrist on the back for 20 times.

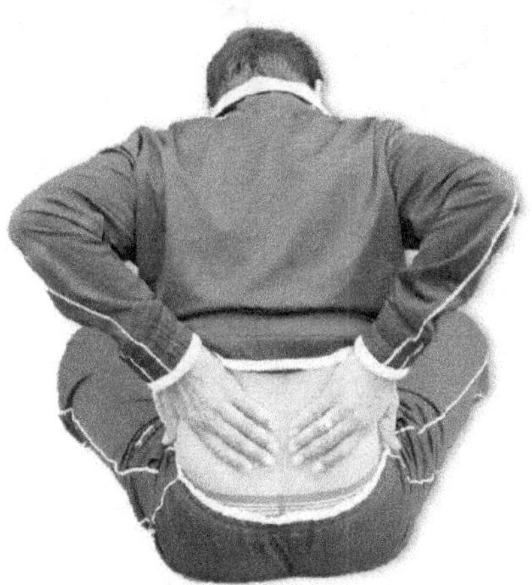

AVII Rub your palms 5 to 10 times and then massage your navel with left hand palm; for women use right hand palm

Do for 1 minute. Please refer the pictures A7 Pic 1 to A7 Pic3

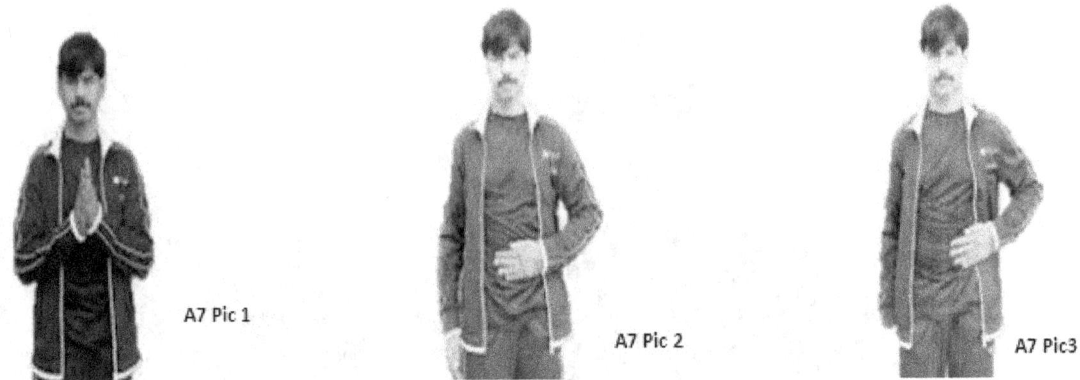

AVIII Massage naval area as show in the picture. This should be done for 1 minute continuously, either in sitting or standing position.

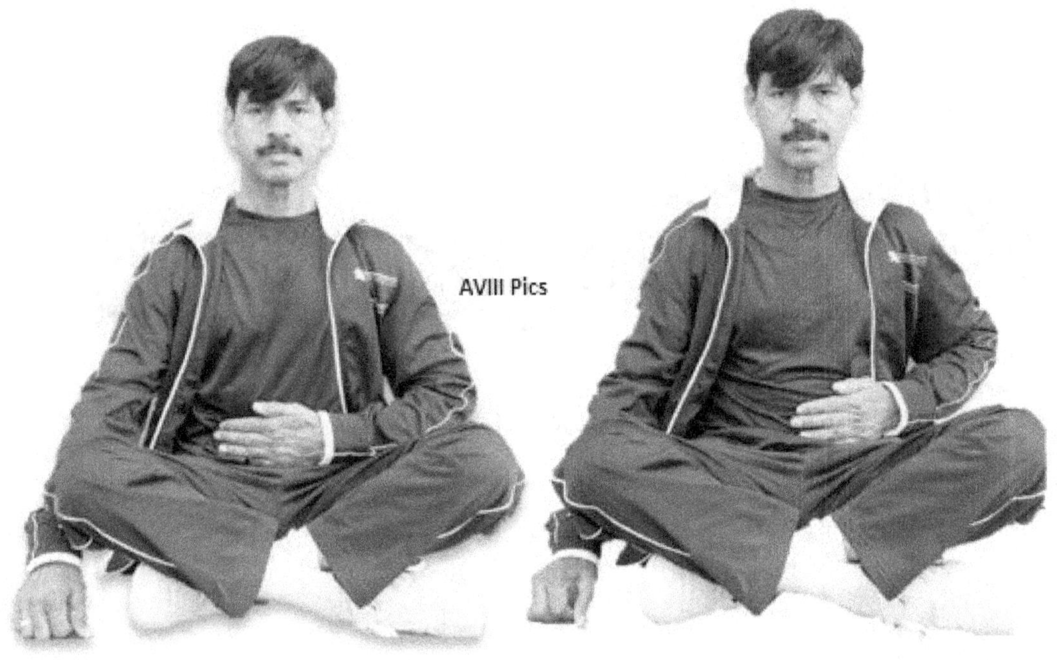

Variation: Stand in horse stance and keep left hand palm on naval and cover with right hand palm and slightly bend upper body and massage clockwise very hard for 10 to 12 times. One should do each movement set 6 times daily.

Massage back (near kidneys) for 1 minute continuously.

AVIII Medicinal exercise
Sit crossed legs and keep hands on knees and rotate your upper body in circular motion. Do this in clockwise for 10 times and anti-clockwise for 10 times.

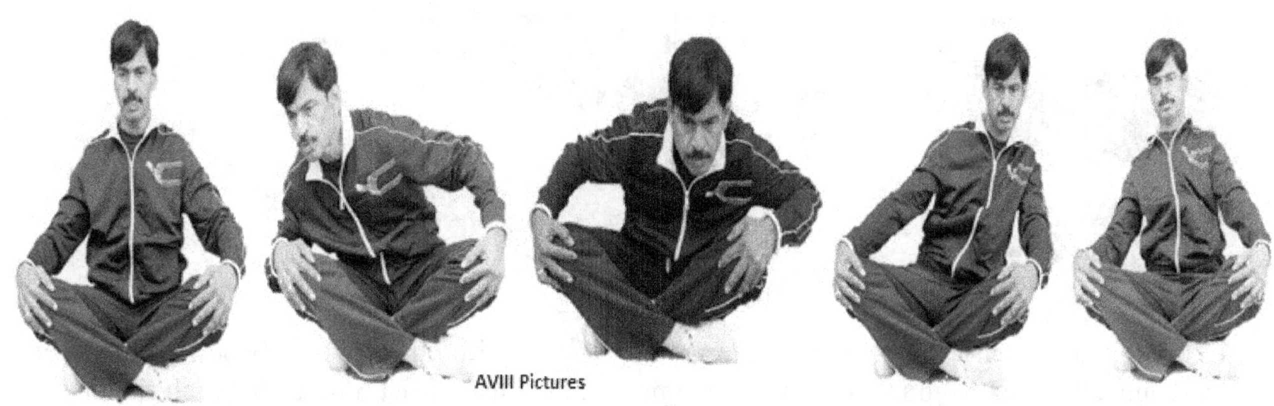

AIX Medicinal Exercise
Drum of Heart or heavenly drums, this exercise stimulates the entire nervous system

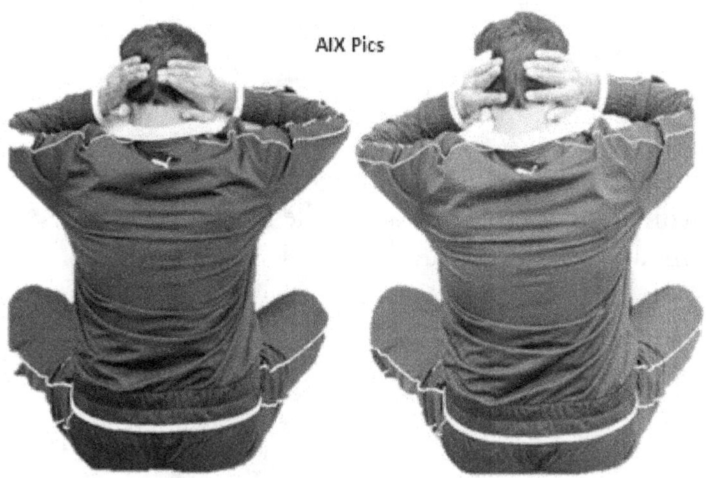

Sit cross legs and close the two ears with palms, keep index finger on the middle finger and hit with the index finger on the skull. This should be done 1 minute continuously. This is also called the Drums of the heart or Drums of heaven. Do this by closing eye and hear the sound of index finger slides off and snaps down on the base of your skull.

AX Medicinal Exercise VIII

Stand and extend right and left hands and palms facing ground and bend thumb slowly up and down and stiffen it. Then gradually bend all fingers one by one. This should be done with breath in and out. One should do this for each finger for 30 secs to 1 minute. This exercise is good for stroke, organ tuning inducing all meridian points.

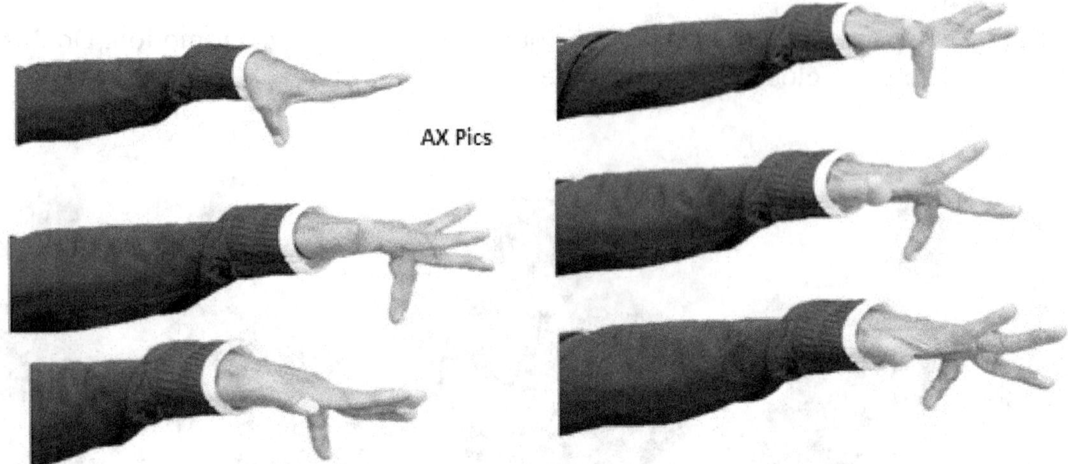

AXI Squeezing each finger with massaging and bending with other hand is beneficial for overall interconnected organs, joints of all meridian points. Do this at least 6 times for each finger

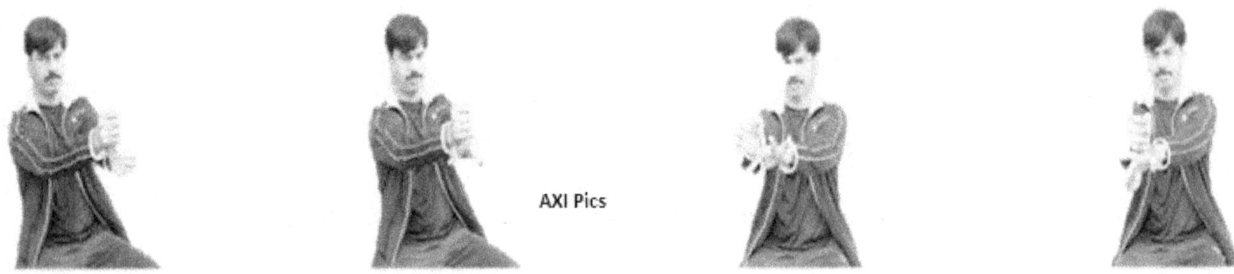

AXII Triple warmer meridian exercise

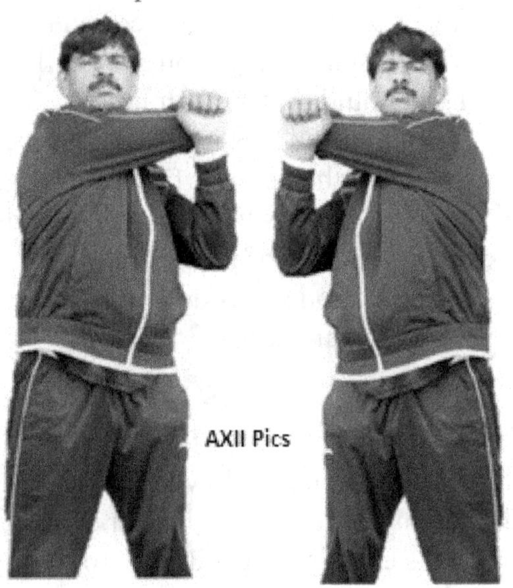

Stand and raise elbow to shoulder level or above like hitting with elbow strike. It is advisable to do this 20 times right and 20 times left.

Medicinal Energy Exercise

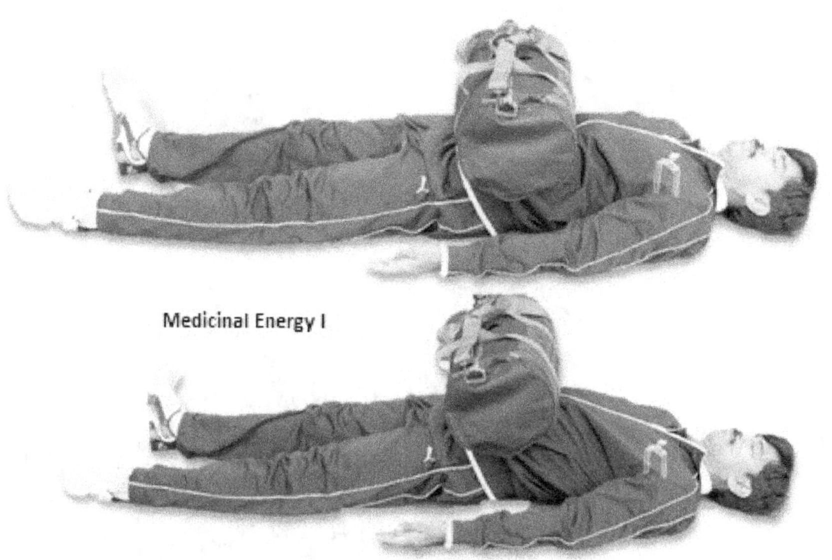

Medicinal Energy I

Medicinal Energy I

Medicinal Energy I

Lie down and keep the hands sideways. Keep a weight of 5 to 8kgs (rectangular bag like rice bag or sand bag) on navel. Breathe in and out with lower abdomen. Push the weight up and bring the bag down, as if you are sleeping. Doing this 5 minutes is very good for overall health and importantly increases Chi energy.

Medicinal Energy II Sit crossing legs, and spinal cord straight with hands in praying position, Breath in from the lower abdomen.
While breathing in, tighten the hands and while breathing out, relax the hands with same position

Medicinal Energy III Sit crossed legs and hands bent at the elbows

Breath in with hands slowly going up. Breath out with hands coming down. See pics below.

Do this for 9 times

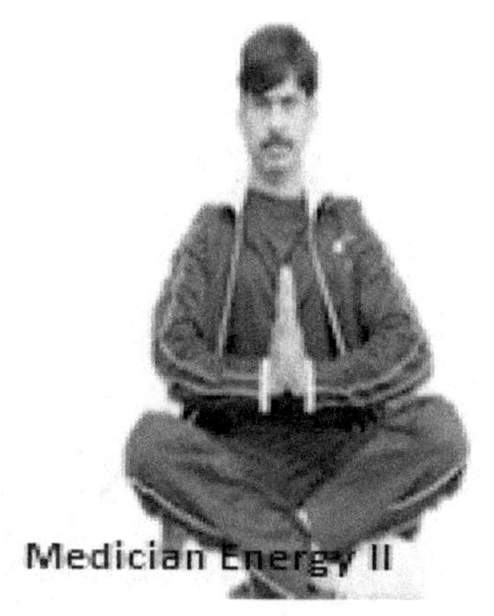

Medician Energy II

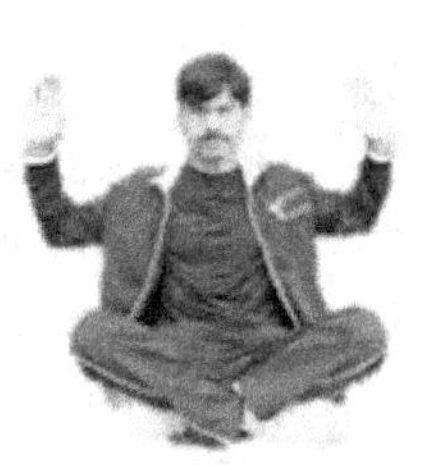
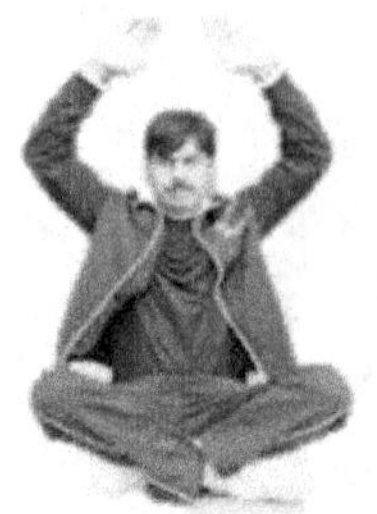
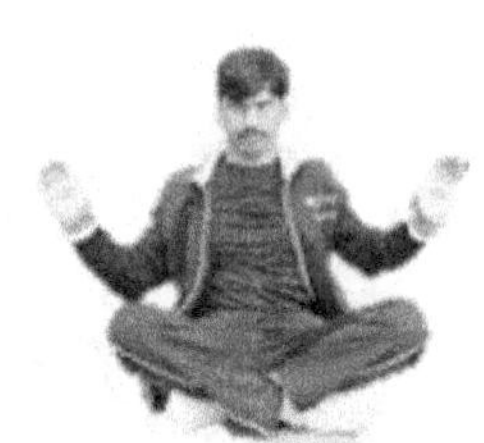

Medicinal Energy III

Medicinal Energy IV Lie down and touch with nose tip to the knee and be there for 10 – 30 secs with lower abdomen stiffened.

Repeat the same with another knee.

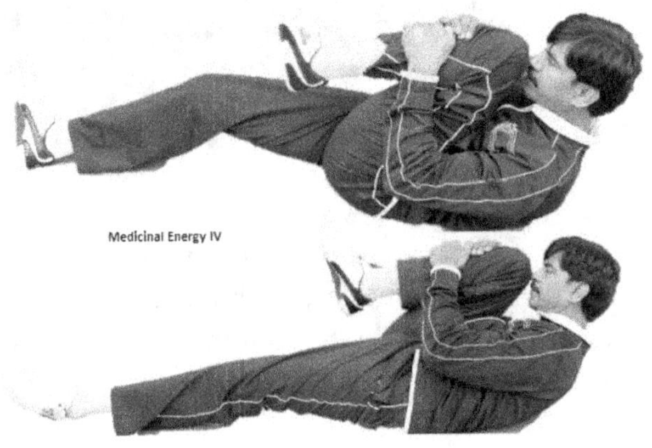

Medicinal Energy IV

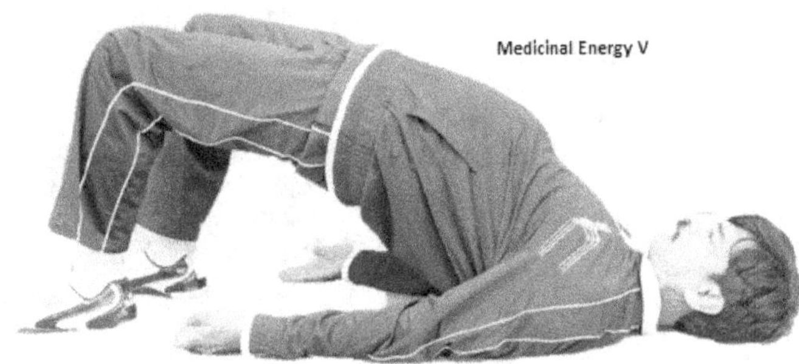

Medicinal Energy V

Medicinal Energy V Lie down, bend your knee and lift your lower back to the maximum and control for 30 seconds. Stiffen your lower abdomen
Repeat the same for two times

VI **Horse** stance and press hands in praying position; breath in and out with standing with hand raising up without separating your hands as shown in the pictures. Again breath in , go on horse stance and breath out while going up with hands in praying position.

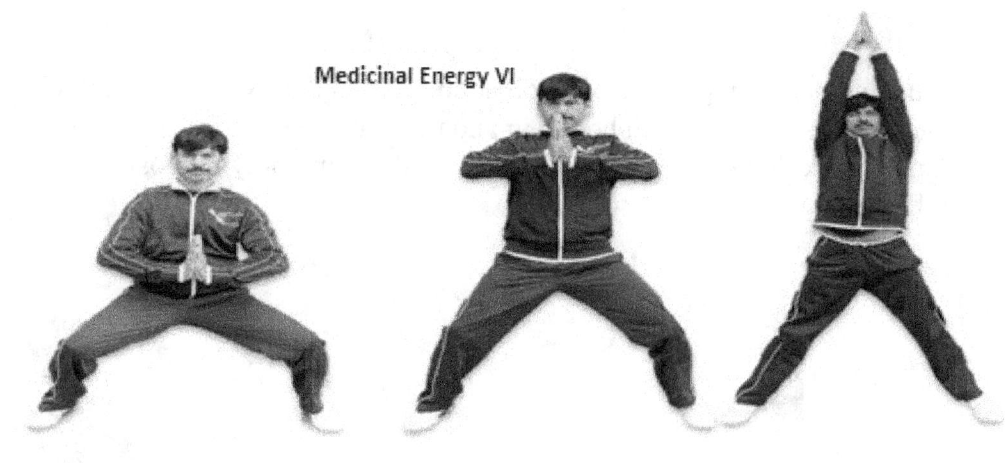

B I

Stand and hands in praying position at chest level and twist your buttocks in the right side and left side. Do this exercise with breath in and out. This exercise is good for all joints, spine, adrenal glands and kidneys. Variation: You can do the same praying position at overhead and twist left and right

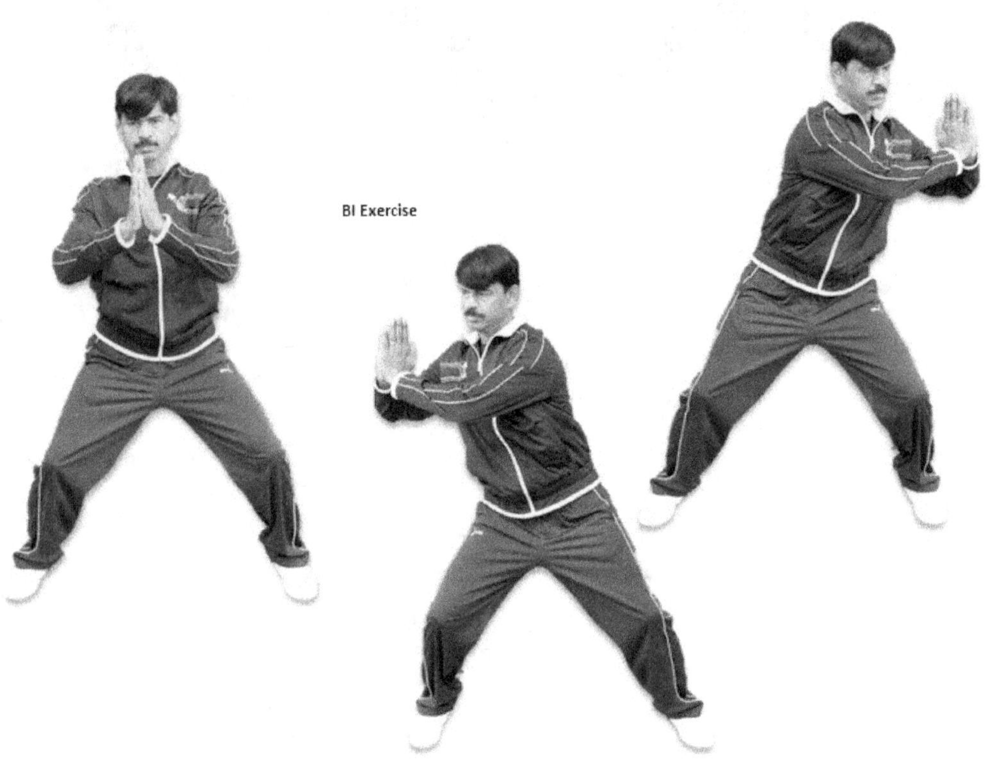

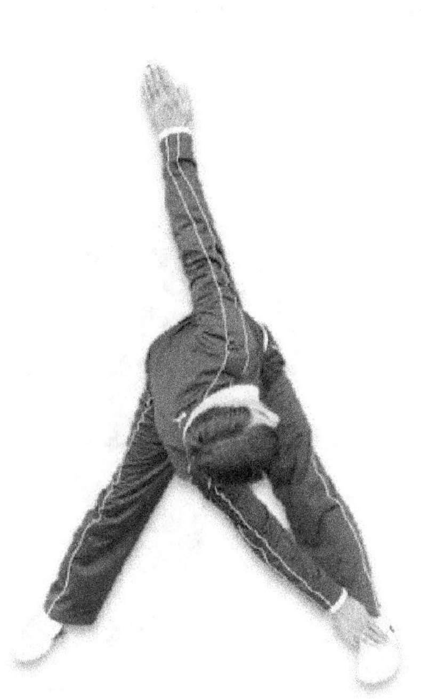

B II Spread your legs and touch the opposite hand and to the toes with other hand while looking straight up sky. Repeat this for 20 times daily. It is very good for brain and spinal cord.

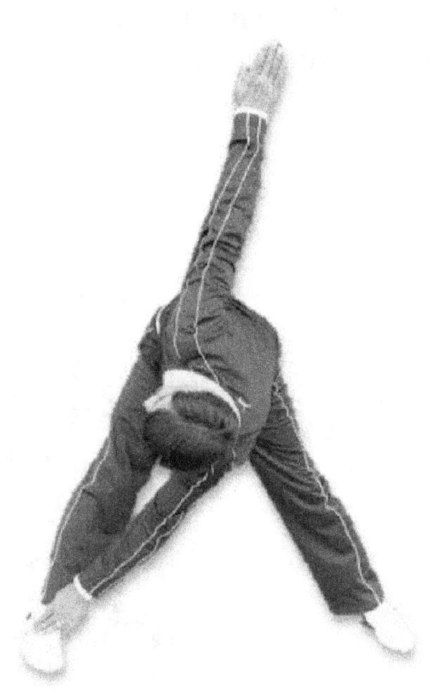

B III Horse stance and spread hands sideways without bending elbows and twist two sides of your body, without moving lower body

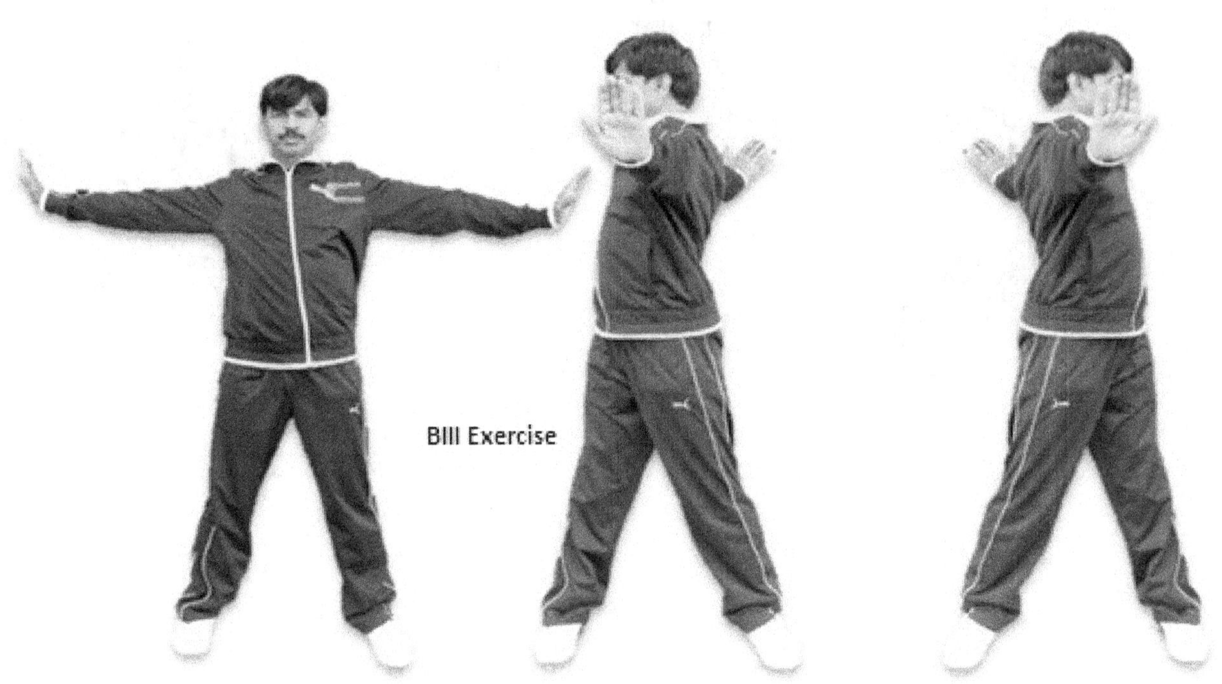

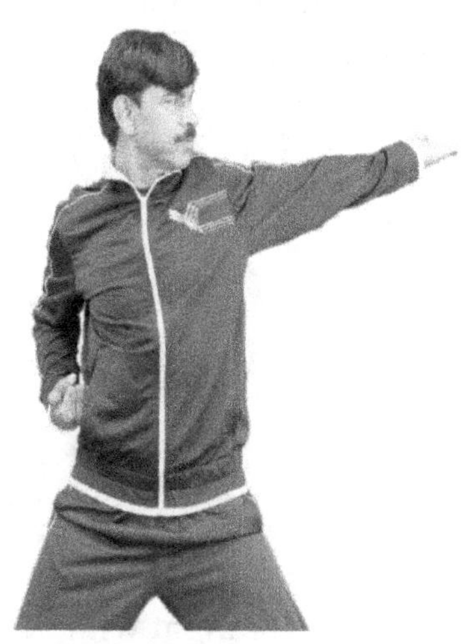 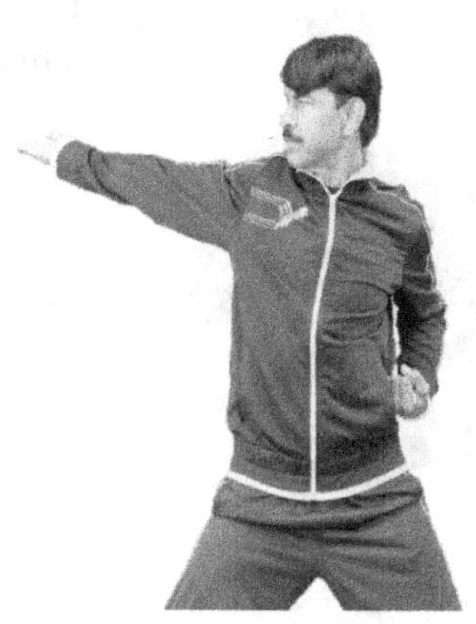

B IV Stand and spread your legs and keep right hand sideways and twisted 180 degrees same side. Spinal cord should be straight and breath out. Do same on the left side. Doing these 10 times each side is very good for brain and pine.

Variation: After you twist the hand in horse stance, you can circulate the hand (6" radius) at the peak twist.

B V Spread legs and twist the body left side with right hand without bending overhead as show in in the picture 1. Doing this exercise 10 times on each side will be beneficial for the gall bladder.

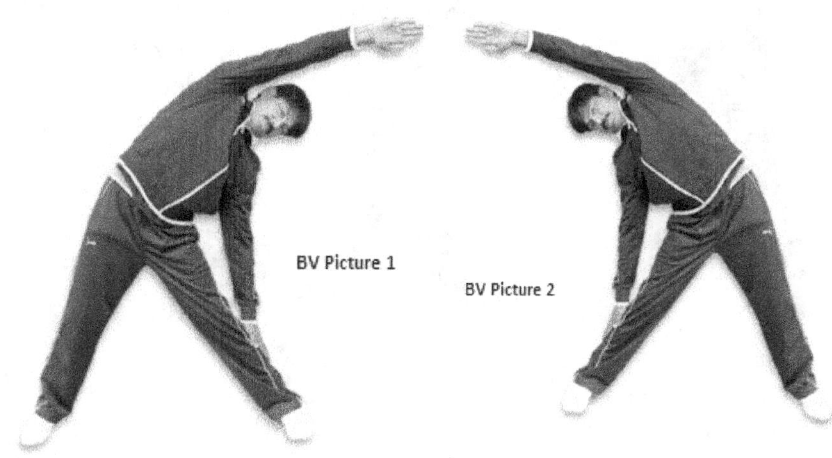

Spread legs , Twist the body towards right and left with hands straight without bending the elbow. Hand and leg should be in single, see picture 2.

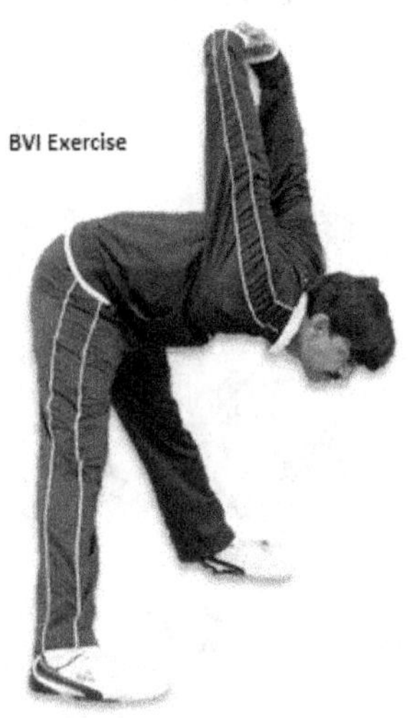

B VI Horse stance and interlock fingers at the back , bend and twist and pull up side with palms facing the sky.
This exercise is good for large intestine.

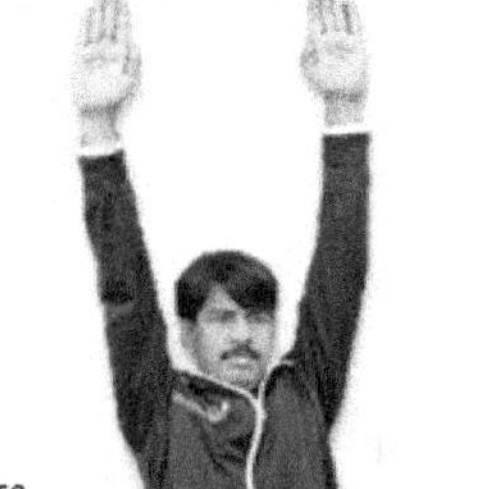

B VII Stand and bring right leg forward straight with hands pulled up straight. Do this exercise alternating left leg forward and vice-versa. Doing this 20 time is very good for spleen and all meridian points related to spine will get activated.

Explanation: Stretching the hands upwards fully and bend the front knee deep stretching, whether you move forward or do at stationary.

B VIII Spread the legs and twist the body left like holding a big wheel to left and right in a circular motion. Do this for 10 times each side.

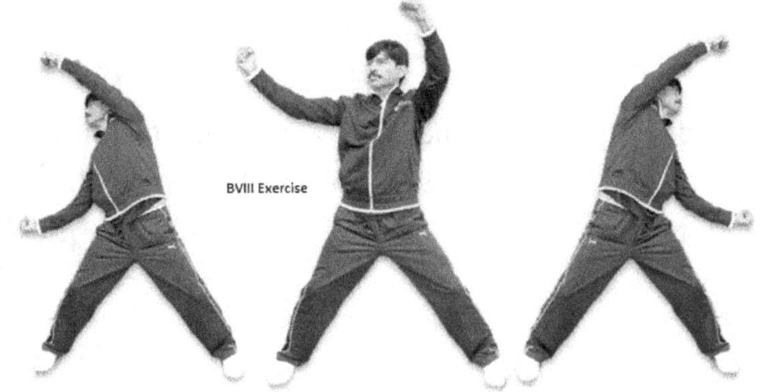

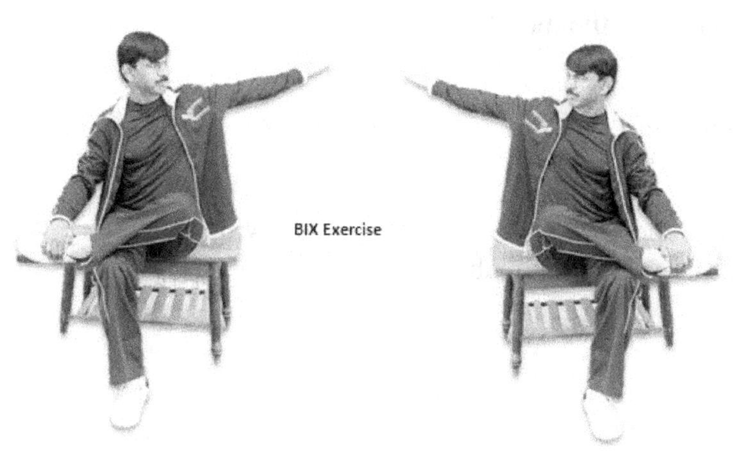

B IX Sit on chair or any platform and put your right leg on the left thigh and extend right hand palms facing the sky. Hold right leg with left hand. Do the same to left side with breath in and extend your arms to maximum back side/twist and breath out, do this exercise for 10 times each side.

B X Stand as if you are holding a big ball and turn the ball with both the hands. First keep the right hand up and left hand down and feel as if you are holding a big ball. Slowly move the hands as if you are rotating the big ball. As you move to the right side, the left hand should come on top.

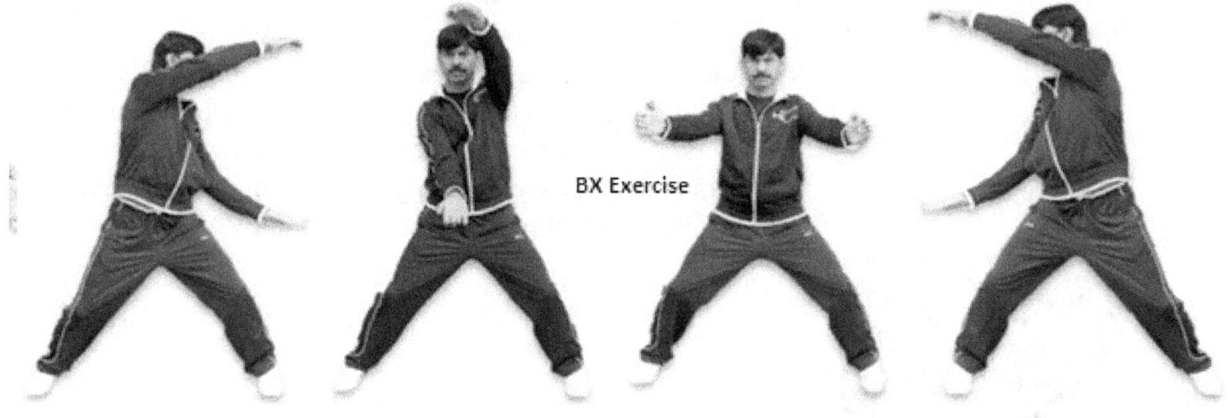

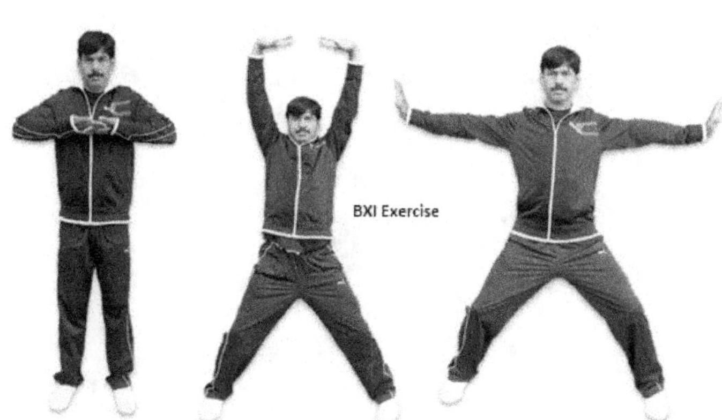

B XI Stand with hands and finger tips facing each other in the front, bring with palms facing the sky near to chest as shown in the picture. Keep breathing till chest and slowly breath out with the hands making a big circle and bring back to side of your thighs as shown in picture. This should be done at least 21 times daily each schedule.

B XII Horse stance and punch slowly with breath out with lower abdomen. Breath in with tongue adhered to roof of the mouth.

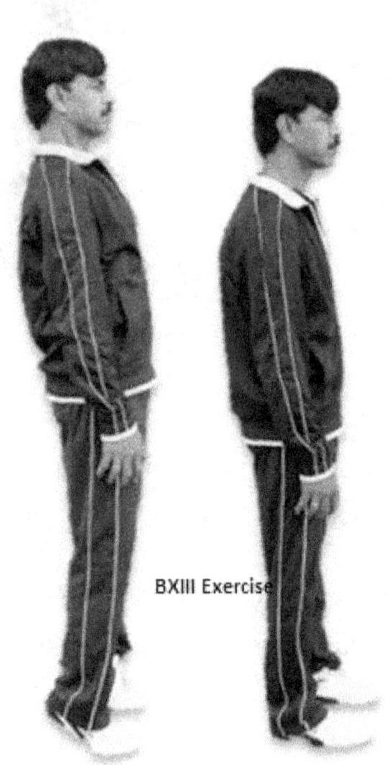

Variations:

1) Punch fast with sound kiai – this is very good for all organs. One should do this for 100 times.

2) Breath in and control for 5 to 10 punches with breath out. Increase daily 10 to 20 punches.

B XIII Energy Jump on toes – Raise feet to 2" to 6" high from the ground and jump. This should be done 50 times every day and is very good for lower body strength.

Note: Aged people who cannot jump, can raise back heel to the ground and bring back to the ground and for others, stand on toes and jerk to come down suddenly as if your whole body is falling on the ground from height. One should do this at least 25 times daily.

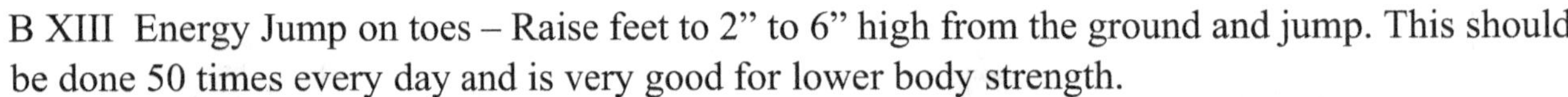

B XIV   Stand and kick to chest level 50 times with right and 50 time with left leg.
This exercise helps to strengthen thighs and also meridian points on thighs.

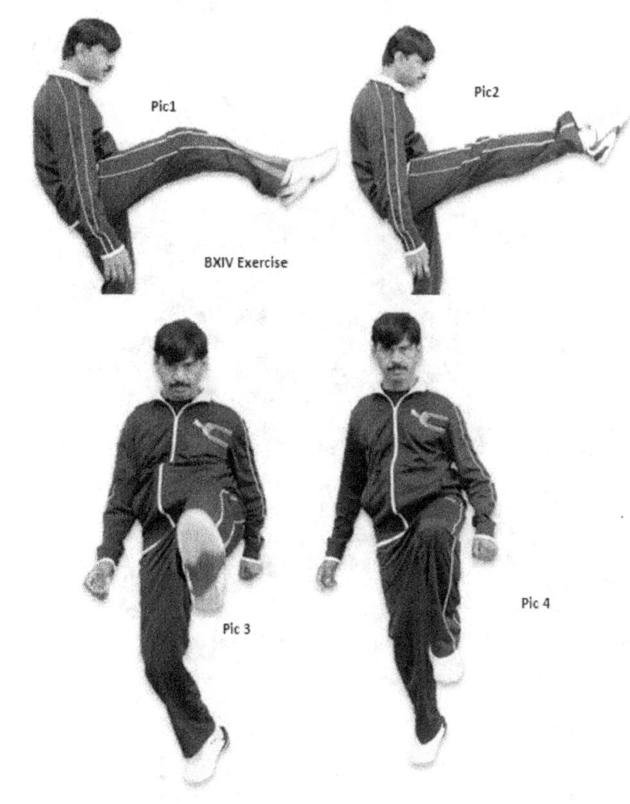

B XV Lie down on palms hands with
shoulder width distance and do push ups
to 15 to 25 times every day.

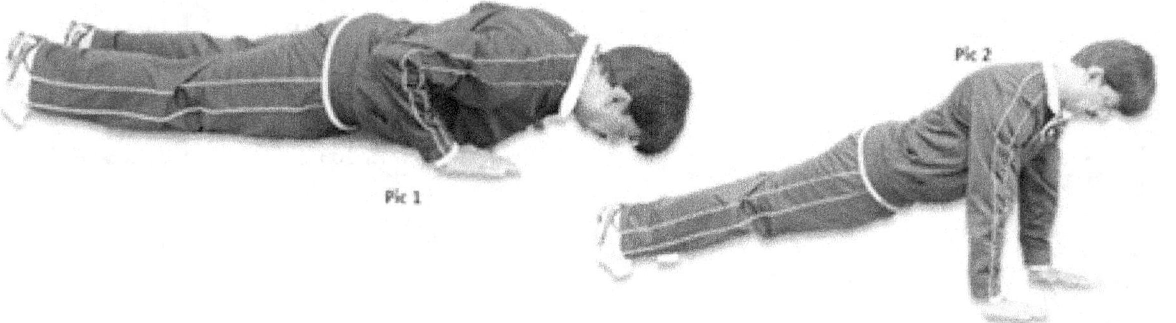

B XVI Squat should be done with knee parallel to ground and upper body should be straight upright. Wall squatting is also best for kidney and overall lower body. Squatting is best exercise, especially for kidneys because the meridian point is located at middle hollow part on the bottom of the foot and continue up through the body on the chest, collar bone etc., which is detailed in the book.

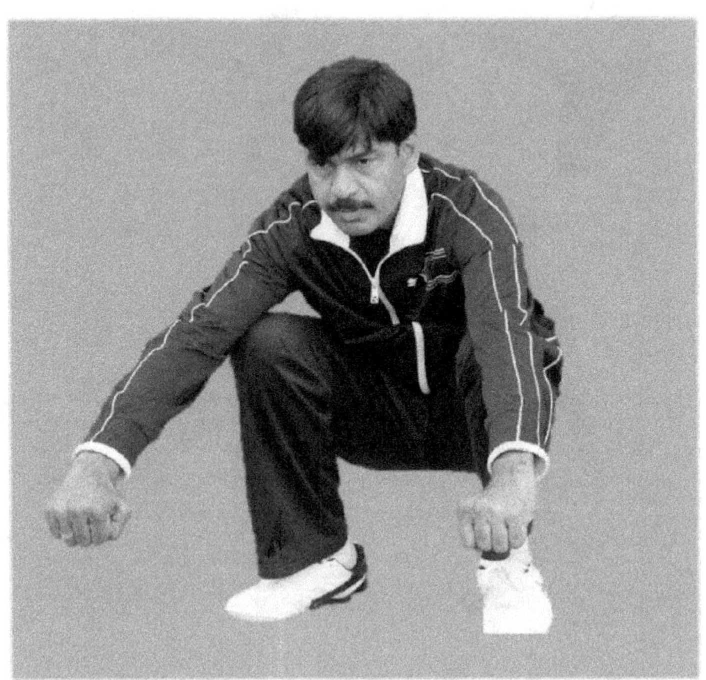

If you do with breathing squats the oxygen circulates throughout kidney meridian pathway from the bottom of the foot to the root of tongue.

Further the kidney meridian moves the energy impulse up into the body and the energy circulated into and through the rest of the meridian.

Squat is the best exercise for lower body, and this was practiced in many parts of the world; this is 2nd only exercise ancient people practiced for almost 3000 years and the first being pushups.

Many physical trainers in the ancient times considered this as king of all exercises.

Various Types of Squats

Hold the 12" to 18" ball above your head with hands straight up and squat with breath out and breathe in while getting up. Breath out while going down. Do at least 10 to 15 times daily

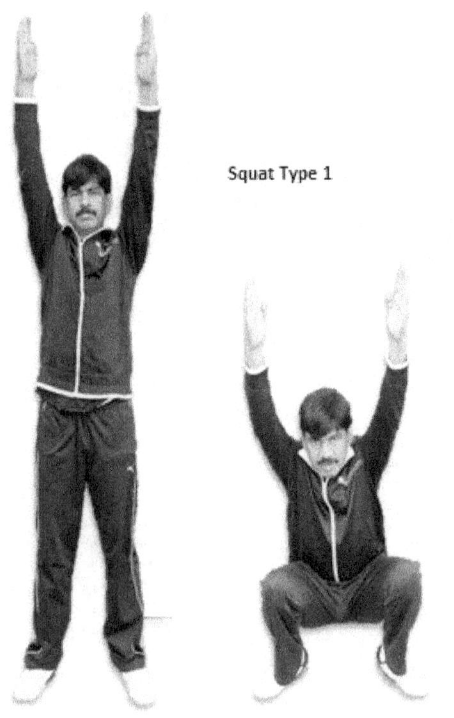

Squat Type 1

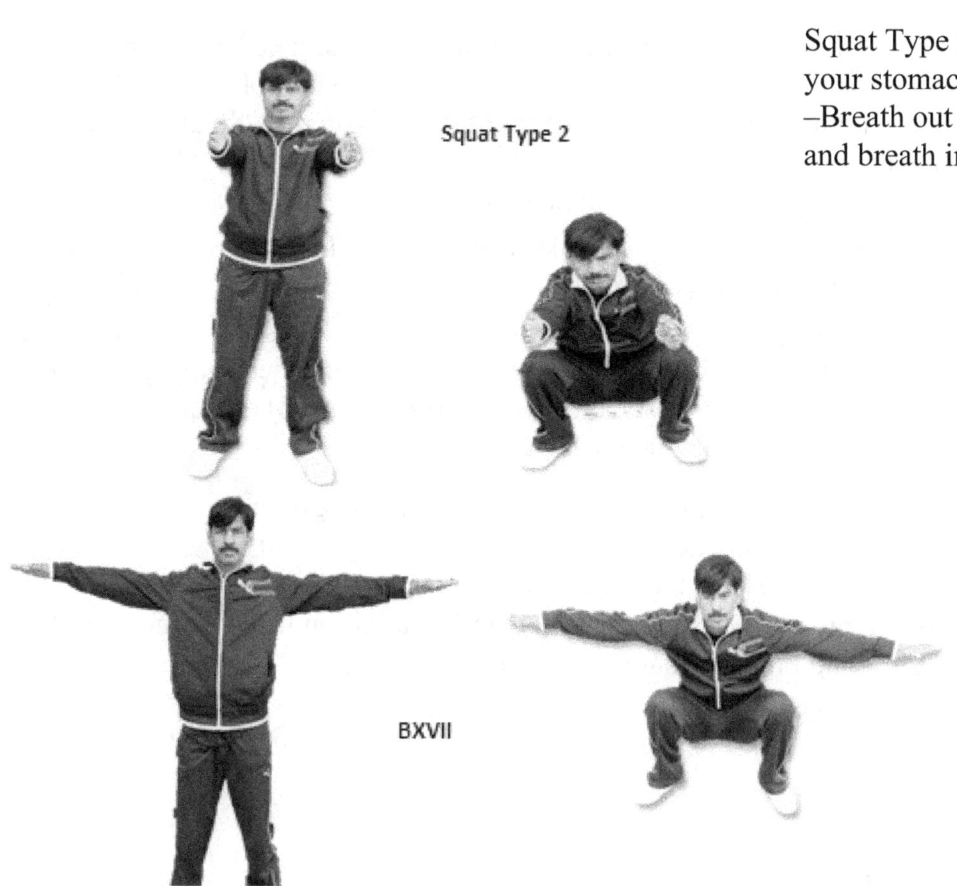

Squat Type 2 : Hold the ball at your stomach level or chest level –Breath out while going down and breath in while raising up

B XVII Hand sideways straight with palms facing the ground – breath out while going down, and breath in while raising up

B XVIII Hand interlock around neck and squat with breath out while going down and breath in while raising up

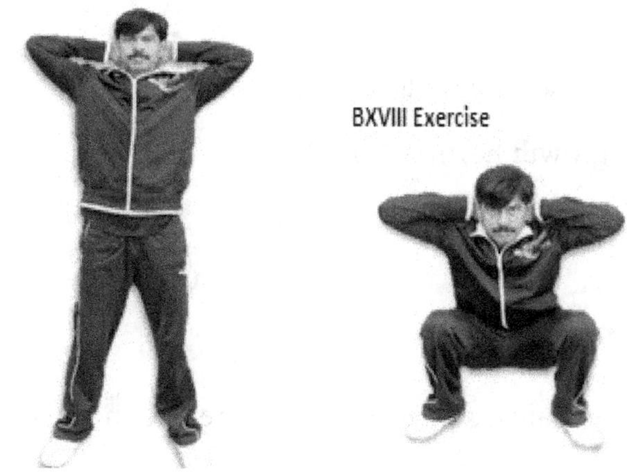

<u>**Variety of Squats**</u>

1. Squatting with partner – If you are not able to squat alone, you can take help from partner. Two partners should stand 2.5 to 3 feet according to your arm's length, facing each other. Squat by balancing each other with hands jointed together at the center. Sit and stand for 20 to 50 times each day.
2. Note: Do not lean in front. Upper body should be straight
3. Squatting with holding edge of the table and squat will help develop your strength in legs initially and later you need to do without support.
4. Squatting with partner – Both partners should stand back to back and see that partners' upper and lower backs are touching each other. Squat with support of each other, go down as low as possible and get up. Doing these 20 times is good for lower body strength and balance. Many martial artists practice this for lower leg strength.

   Note: All the above Squats should be done with thighs parallel to ground and head, back and spinal cord in a straight line.

Squat is a miracle exercise and it moves and strains every meridian point of the body. Key benefits are – helps circulate impulses to all the meridian points in addition helps oxygenates the blood and moves the oxygen through the circulatory system of all meridians.

There are several benefits in squats including

Cardiovascular health,

Balance,

Endurance, strength, and stability,

Leg strength,

Prevent osteoporosis,

Increases bone density

Metabolizes nutrition to all tissues, glands and colons

Increases testosterone and growth hormone production

Prevents inflammatory bowel syndrome

Efficient digestion

Helps faster weight loss

Apart from the above gains, squats also help strengthen spinal muscles, quadriceps, calf muscles, and hamstrings.

I hope you follow the instructions on how to do various types of Squats. Start with 10 a day and increase to 40 to 50 per day. One can start doing the squats 10 in the morning and 10 evening till you get strength in your legs and move on to do 50 squats at one stretch per day.

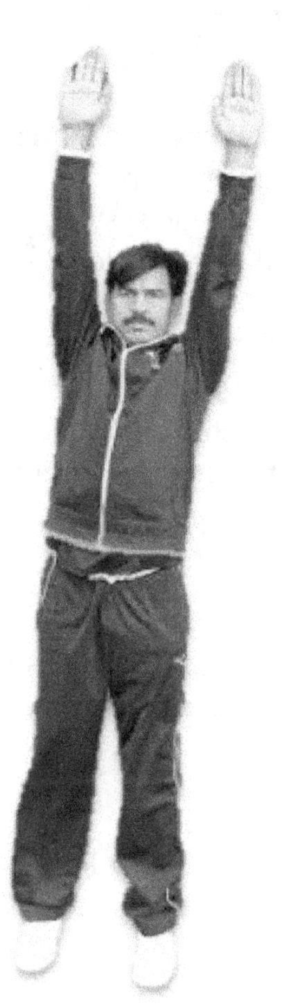

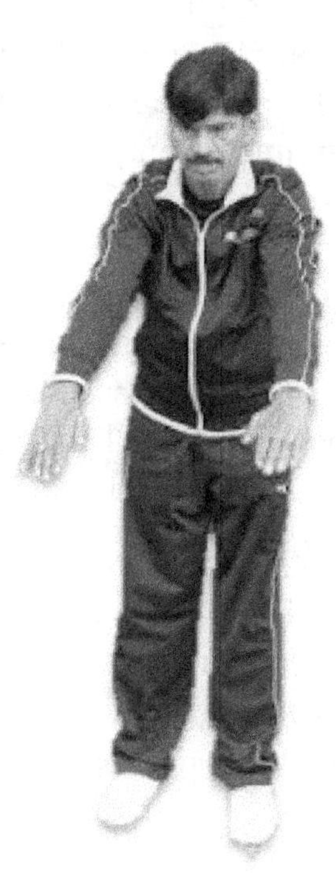

B XIX
Stand straight and raise hands up with heels also raised along with breath in and breathe out, by bringing the hands down with feet flat on the ground and bend a little upper body with each breath in and out. This should be done in open area where lot of trees/plants are surrounded.

Note: While breath out bring your hand down, do fast breath out with sound HUWWWWW.

B XX Stand straight and bend forward by touching the toes with your fingers (raising your toes while holding).
These exercises are advised to be done 6 to 12 times daily

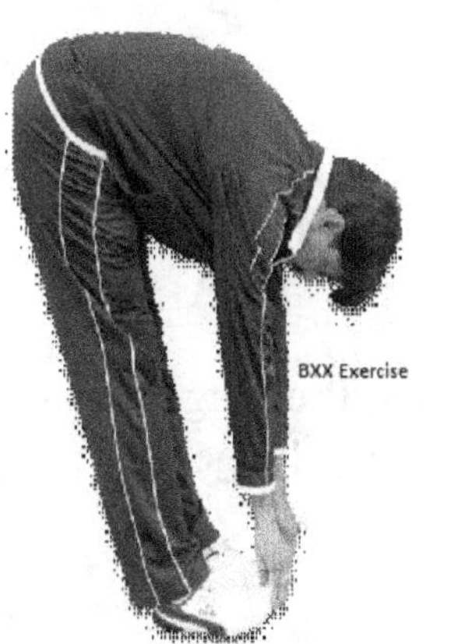

Kidney Meridian

This point is on the sole of your feet. It is center of your sole on two legs. Press hard to that point for a minute and release. This will help kidney to heal. This point is very important because it can stimulate your entire nervous system and wake up especially your endocrine system and helps to improve your circulation. This helps blood flow to your pelvic cavity and helps to slowdown aging process.

Spleen Meridian/Stomach

Sit down and cross your legs one over the other so that your top leg is at a 90degree angel. Using ankle bone as a straight point from there, 4 inches on the side of the shin bone. Pressing that point hard for 1 minute and releasing will help solve reproductive problems, spleen and many important connected meridian points.

Large Intestine Meridian

This point is located between your thumb and your index finger. Open your thumb and index finger wide. Do you see a V shape? At the edge of that V press gently at that point for 1 minute on each side. This is good for immune system, relieves pain – pelvic pains, headache, and helps keep healthy nervous system and all connected meridians.

Multiple Organ Golden Point

This point is at below the knee. There is nose like bone besides that points. You can press hard on both the legs at this point for – strengthening of legs. In ancient times, monks and yogis used to walk hundreds of miles by pressing that point whenever they were tired.

Diamond Point

Diamond Point is located midway between your anus and genitals. Put or keep a small bouncing ball on the point and sit. You can sit on chair and keep for 10 minutes. There are many meridians connected to this point and will give healing effect on reproductive organs.

Skull and Pituitary gland

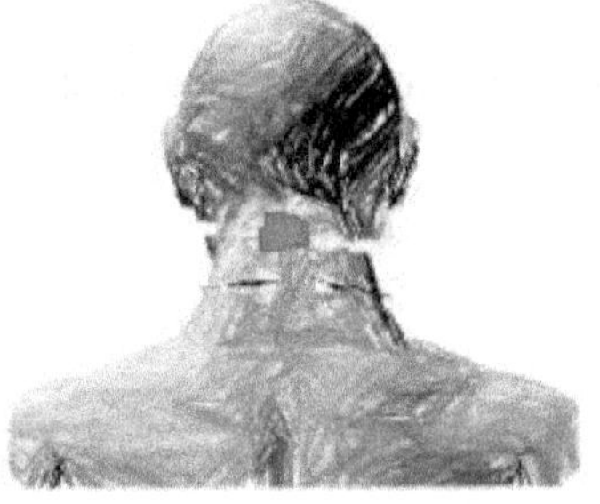

Press at the base of the skull and center at pituitary gland.

Forearm

The point on right forearm which is 3" inches from elbow is sore point. Pressing it for 1 minute everyday gives us healing effect on all organs and thereby helping longevity

Navel

Press navel with middle finger and breathe in and breathe out. Relax. Doing this for 1 minute will help all organs immensely.

Mouth

Open mouth and place thumb on inside of middle of left cheek with forefinger on outside of same spot and pinch gently but firmly; hold for 6 seconds. Do the same on the right cheek as well. This will relieve stress, tension, anxiety etc.,

Eye Brows

Press eyebrows with thumb bone or index finger knuckle for 1 minute

Centre of mustache

Press with index finger on center of mustache and press center of lower lip below Chin bone.

Advanced Medicinal Martial Yoga Exercises

In this Martial Yoga the crucial rule of the body is hips. The hips are engine through which our body moves; it controls and balances your ability to sit, stand, twist, reach, bend, walk, stepping and running etc., Everything goes through the hips including all meridian acupressure points. Hip muscle attaches to vertebra of the lower spine. Hips connects to a tandem and attaches to the diaphragm and it connects to your breathing and upon it sits all the major organs.

Think of this as a barometer which is an indicator of the health and strength of your whole body. The hidden most powerful survival tool is the hip muscle. When the hip muscle is healthy – we are healthy. Hips are bridge between your upper body and lower body. They are the center of your body's movement. If we are not conditioning the hips, we are inviting problems – primarily joint pains in legs, lower back pain, discomfort while walking, bad posture, trouble sleeping, high anxiety, digestive problems, compromised immune system, circulatory problems, loss of sexual performance, lack of explosiveness in all sports including martial arts.

So, take precaution – and prevention of hip problems is the key and conditioning the hip is the solution. The below mentioned martial yoga will do justice to hips and will help in overall body health and longevity.

Advanced Medicinal Martial Yoga 1) Sit cross legs and take left hand, cover your right ear – breath in with nose slowly, while keeping the tongue adhered to the top of the mouth for 15 to 20 secs.

Breath out slowly with mouth.

Do it at least for 3 mins to 5 minutes (Pic1)
Change the other hand and repeat the same for 3 to 5 minutes (Pic2)

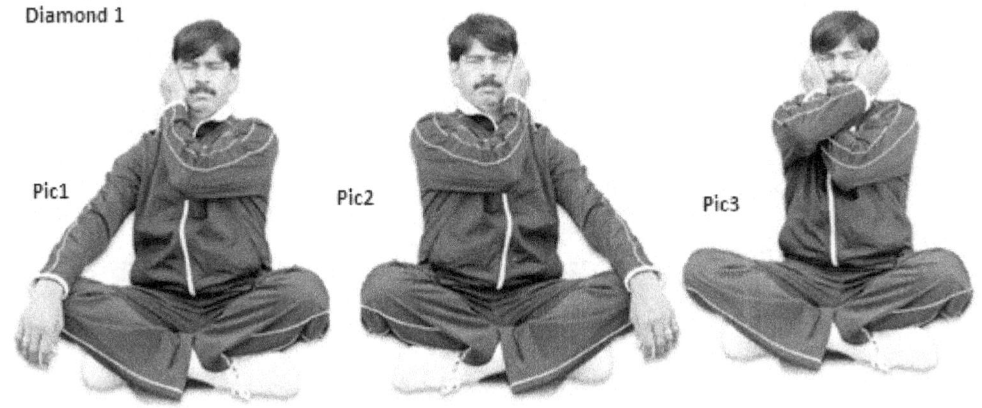

Change by putting left hand on right ear and right hand over left ear and breath in slowly and breath out slowly. Take 15 to 20 secs each breath. Do for 3 to 5 minutes (Pic3).
Note: This breath in and out must be done with eyes closed.

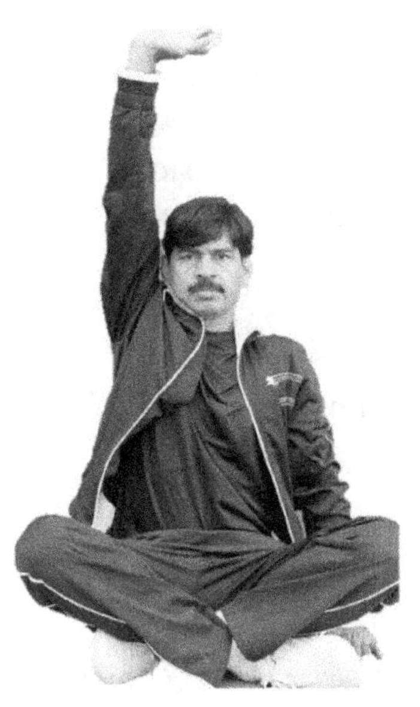

Advanced Medicinal Martial Yoga II Sit crossed legs, raise your left palm sky facing and press the right palm on the ground. Breath in from lower abdomen and control maximum time and breath out. Repeat with other hand also for 5 times each.

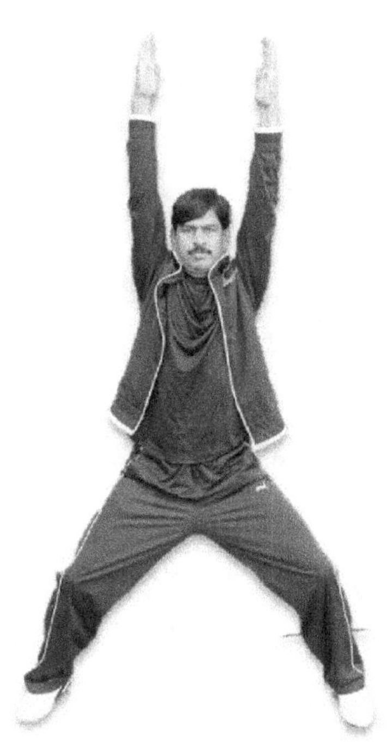

Advanced Medicinal Martial Yoga III

Horse stance with double the shoulder distance between the legs

Hands stretched upwards with fingers facing the sky

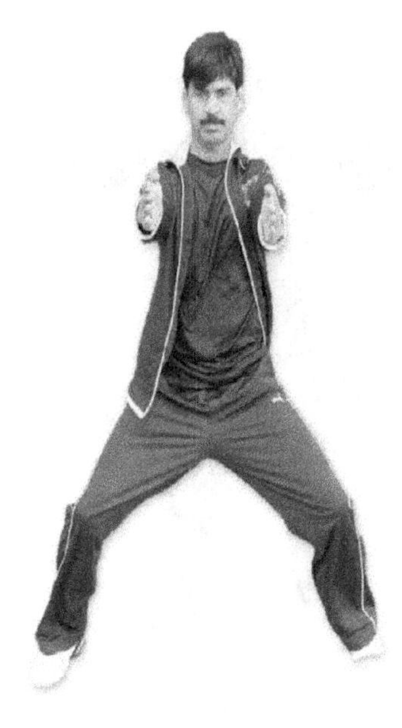

Breath in and out from the lower abdomen, repeat for 5 times

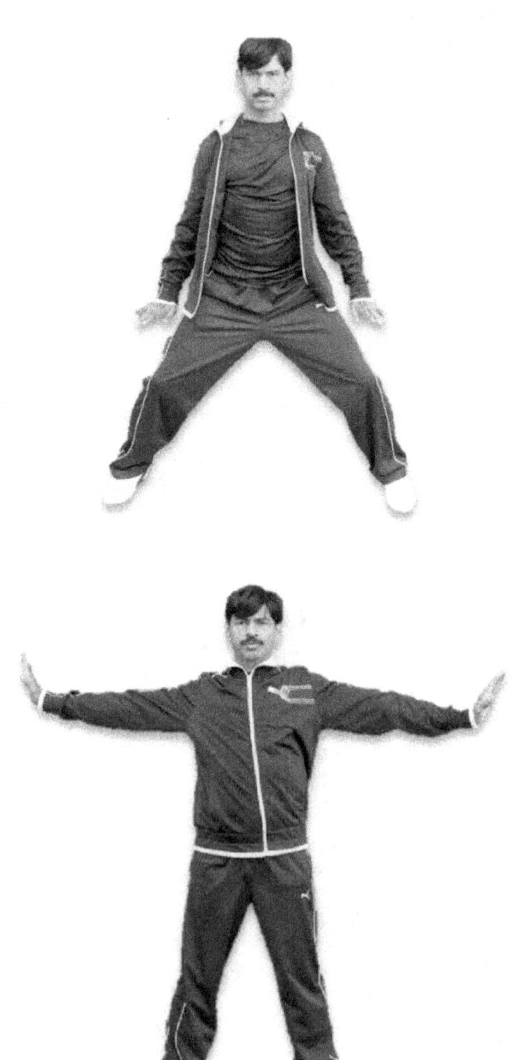

Advanced Medicinal Martial Yoga IV **Horse** stance with double the shoulder distance between the legs.

Hands pressed down.

Breath in from abdomen with hands stretching down.

Breath out slowly from lower abdomen.

Advanced Medicinal Martial Yoga V **Horse stance** with double the shoulder distance between the legs Hands pressed sideways
Breath in from abdomen and
Breath out slowly from lower abdomen. Relax!

Advanced Medicinal Martial Yoga VI Rotate your right foot with left hand. Do 10 times clockwise and 10 time anti clockwise.
Repeat the same for left foot and right hand.

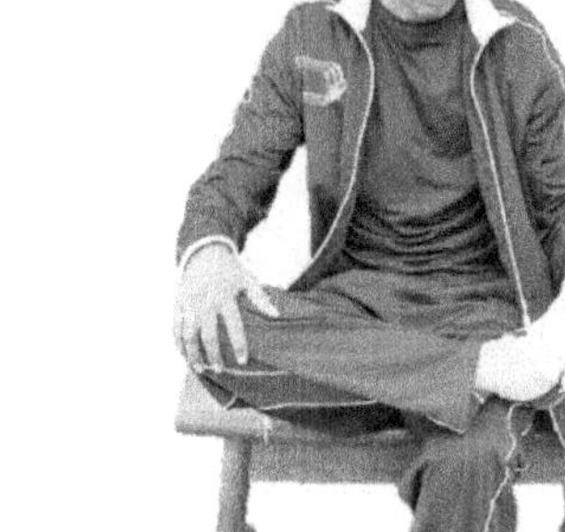

Advanced Medicinal Martial Yoga VII

Walk on knees like a kid.

This exercise is very good for ligaments.

Every day you should do for at least one minute.

Crawling is the best exercise for strengthening the knees, neck, shoulders and good for rehabilitation after stroke, joint injuries, surgery. Crawling directly exercises many muscles groups of lower and upper body. The body of human is meant for four-legged walk: after evolution from animal to human, people started walking on two legs – from ape to super ape. This two-legged walking damages knees and hips because the gravity of earth pulls our upper

Crawling

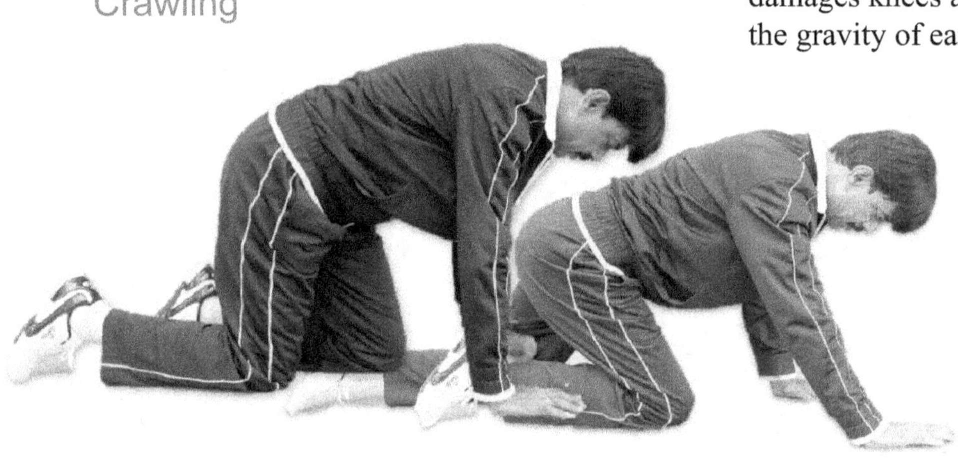

body
downwards,
thereby putting
extra weight legs
and strains on
organs through
the meridian
points from hips

and knees and damages health. So that's why at least crawling a few steps will eradicate many problems. God already trained animals and humans on how to treat various diseases – he made both human beings and animals walk on bare foot. One can see animals putting two hands and two legs to walk and move forward. There are several meridian points related to organs in palm and foot, which get activated during crawling. The meridian points get impulses to the connected organ and makes animals disease free. So, the same way, if a person crawls with palms and foot touching the ground, the meridian points associated with the organs will send impulses to the respective organ and will keep us healthy and happy.

Note: People with knee problems can do this on the mat.

Advanced Medicinal Martial Yoga VIII) **Lock your hands and without bending knees rotate the hands towards your front and touch your feet.**

Do at least 5 times slowly clockwise and anti-clockwise. Refer the pictures below.

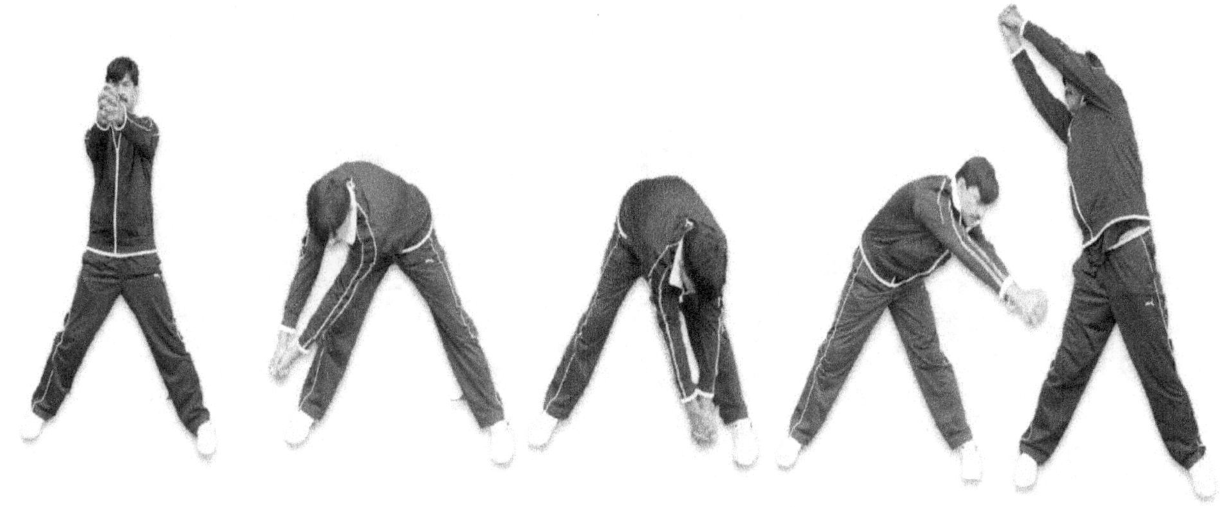

Advanced Medicinal Martial Yoga IX) **Like the previous exercise, do this time on the side of your body**

Legs with double shoulder width.

Shake your hands and legs vigorously for 30 secs.

Repeat for 2 times.

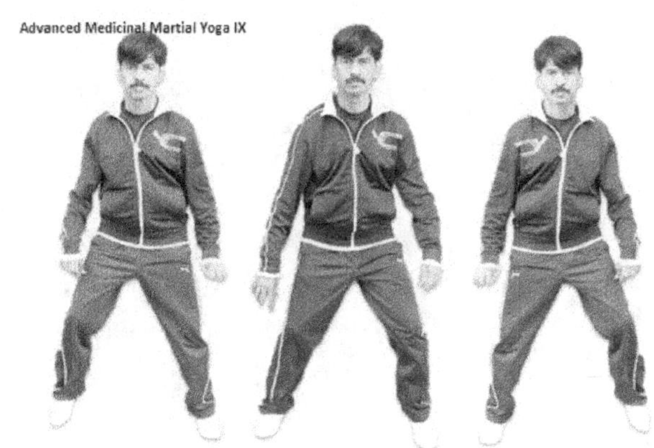

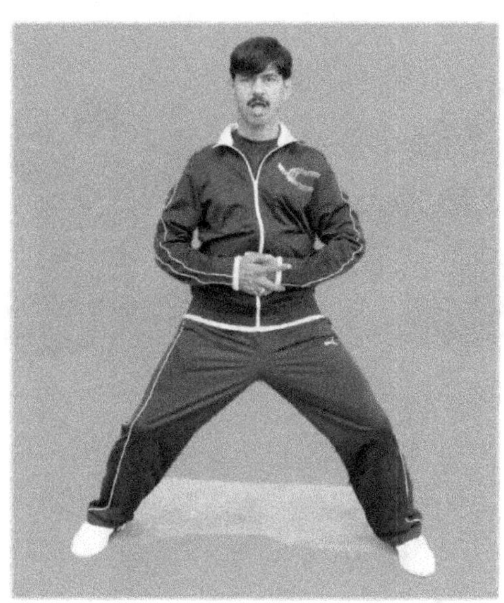

Advanced Medicinal Martial Yoga X) **Stand with knees bent.**

Press your navel with your left palm.

Cover your left palm with you right palm.

And press hand to the stomach.

Breath out with the sound "Howww" .

While breathing out with Howww sound, slightly bend your knees down.

Advanced Medicinal Martial Yoga XI) **Squat sit,**

Hold your feet with hands, stand up.

Twist buttocks and hips to either side like tail for 5 to 7 times.

This is very good for all your ligaments.

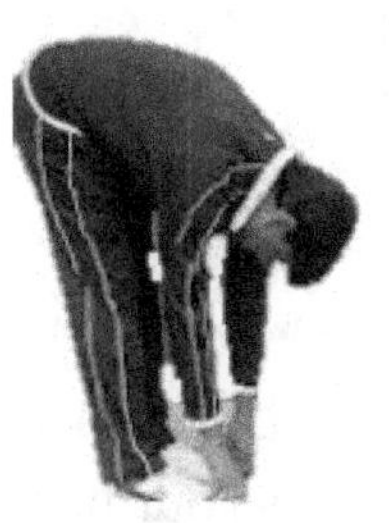 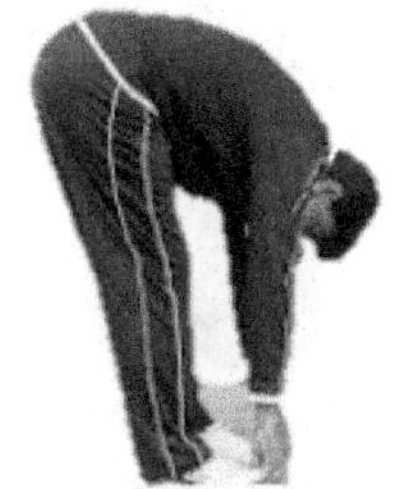 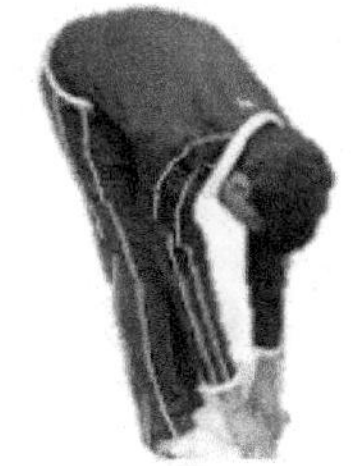

Advanced Medicinal Martial Yoga XII) **Lie down on back,** raise your hands and legs – shake your hands and legs like a crying baby.

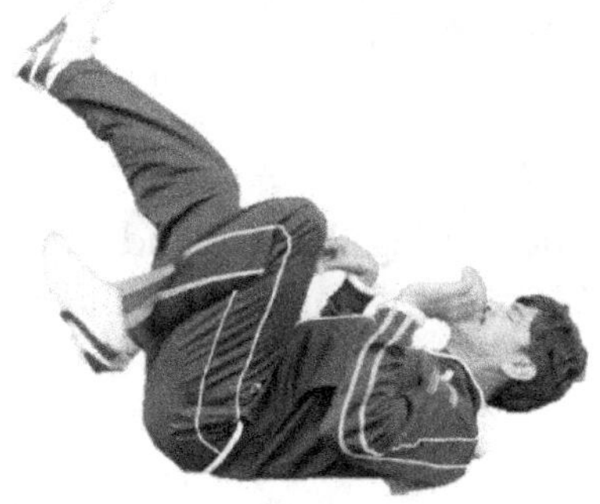

Advanced Medicinal Martial Yoga XIII) **Sit crossed legs and interlock your fingers**

Place your
hands on the
skull

Bend
left
and right to
the maximum
like a
swinging
pendulum.

Do it for 20 times.

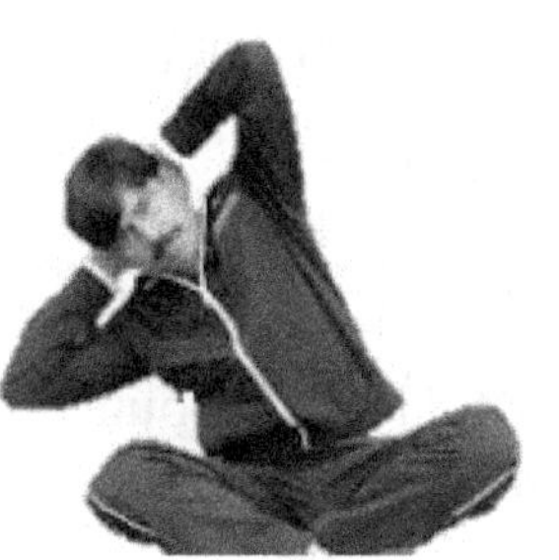
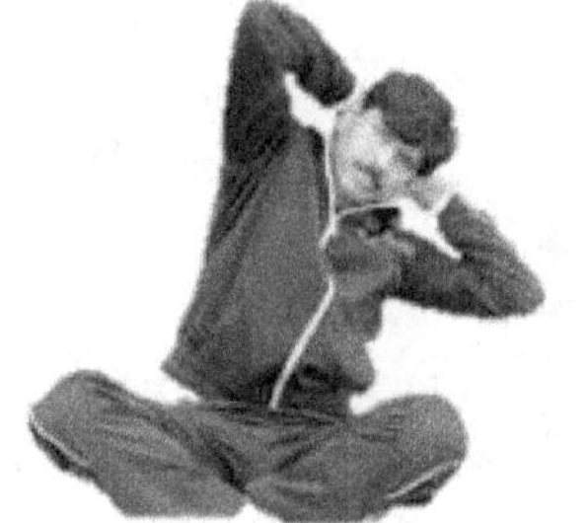
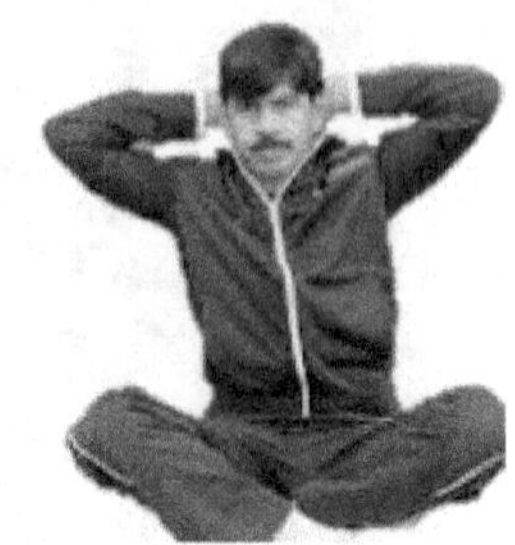

Advanced Medicinal Martial Yoga XIV) **Sit on**
the left leg.
Right leg extended.
Extend your hands backwards.
Swing your hands to front and back with breath
in and out. Do it for 10 times.
Change the legs and repeat the same.

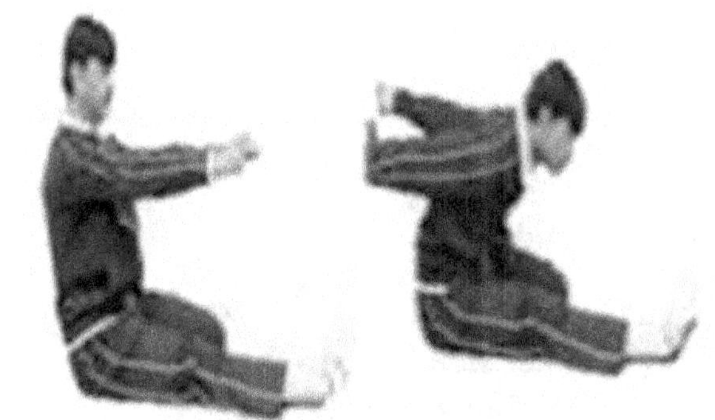
Advanced Medicinal Martial Yoga XIV

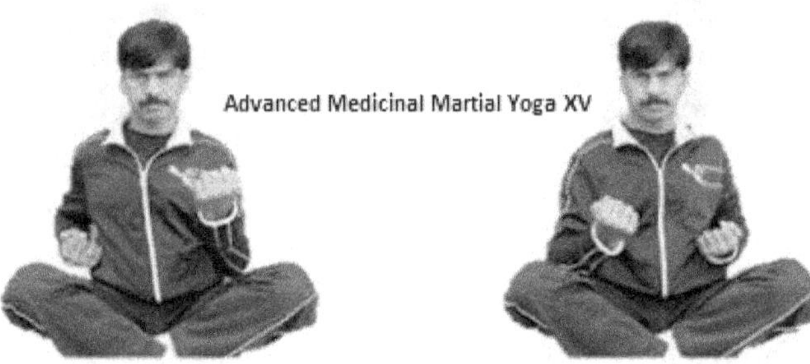
Advanced Medicinal Martial Yoga XV

Advanced Medicinal Martial Yoga XV) **Sit crossed**
legs and swing your hands on the sides front and
back like a half punch, do it for half a minute daily.

Advanced Medicinal Martial Yoga XVI) **Stand right leg perpendicular to**
the left leg. Right hand extend front, move the hand to the back side.
Repeat the same with other hand.
Do it for 5 times each hand.

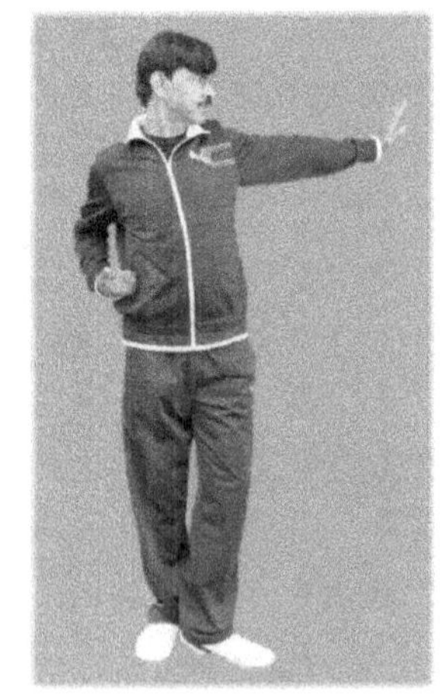

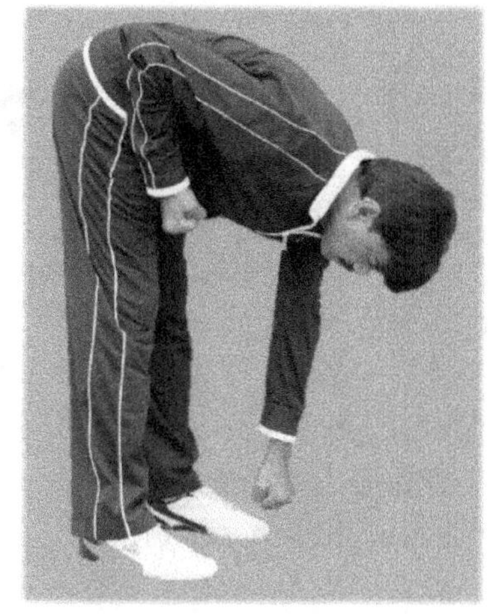

Advanced Medicinal Martial Yoga XVII Stand and bend your body front. Do punches to the ground for 30 times.

Advanced Medicinal Martial Yoga XVIII) Sit with the legs e x t e n d e d . T a

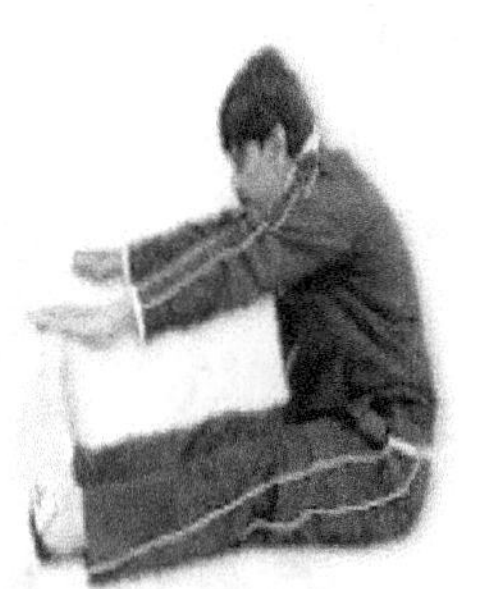 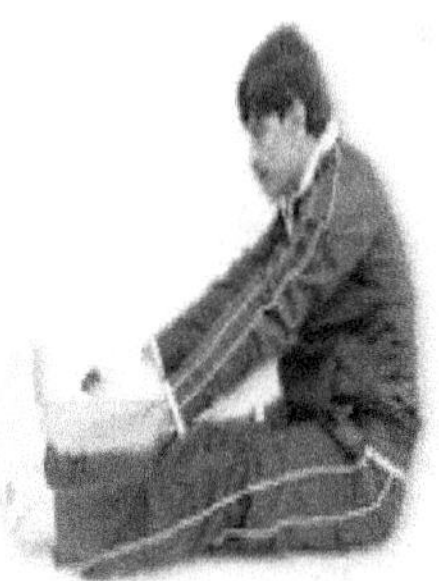 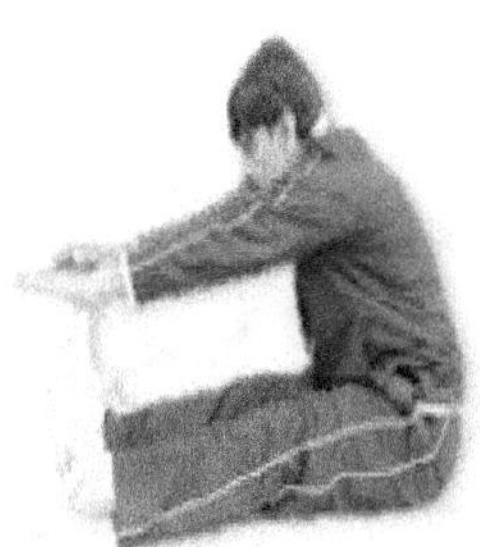 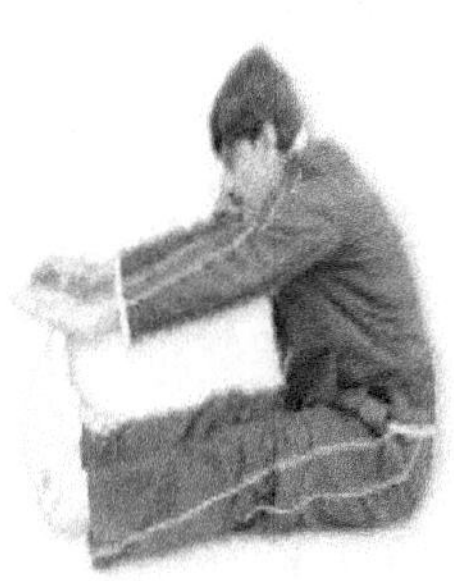 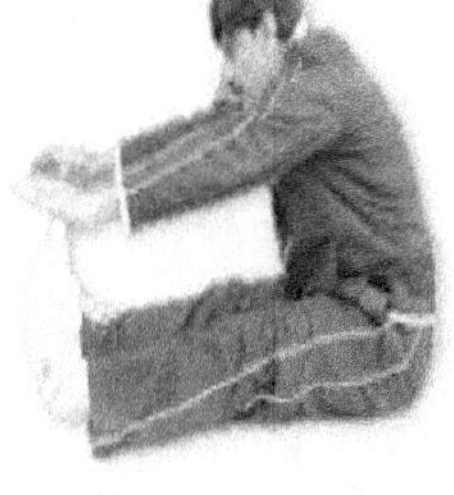

ke out your hands and move your hands over toes in a circular way. Do it for 10 times clockwise and anti-clockwise.

Advanced Medicinal Martial Yoga XIX) Lie down in push up position and do peddling. In this exercise you should bring your knees to your chest level and draw back like peddling.

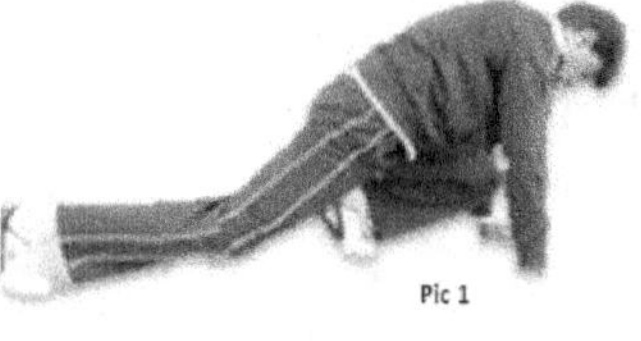

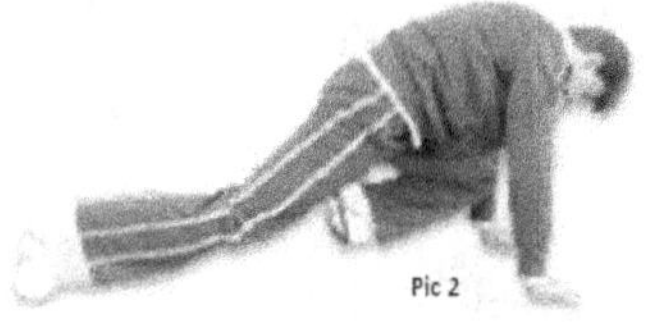

Advanced Medicinal Martial Yoga XX) **Lie down in push up position.**
Pull your two legs to the chest level. And draw back faster.
Do it for 30 times a day.
Please see pics 1, 2 and 3.

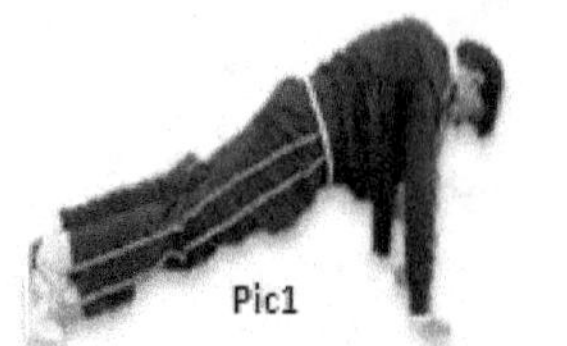

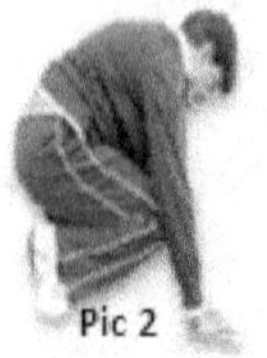

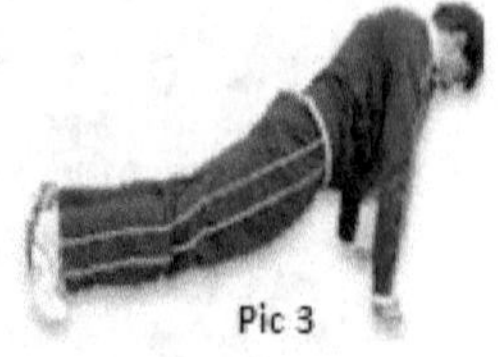

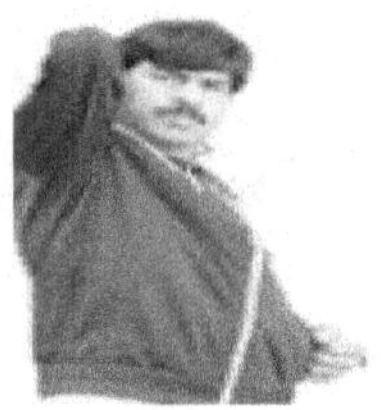

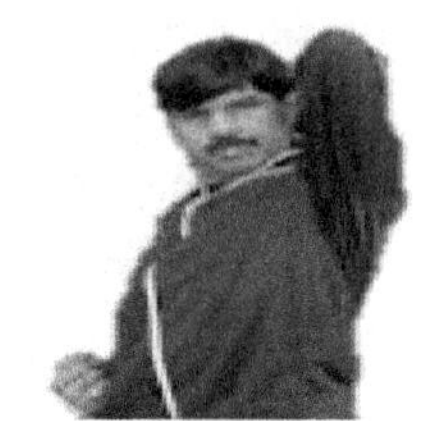

Advanced Medicinal Martial Yoga XXI **Stand and bend your right elbow and hit at your face level**

Do the same with left elbow - Do 10 to 20 times each

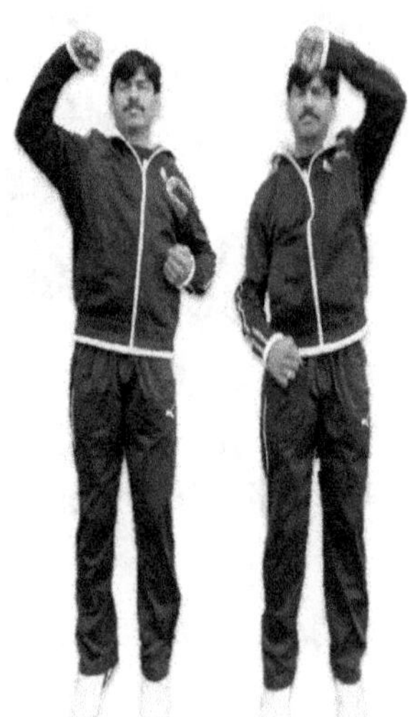

Advanced Medicinal Martial Yoga XXII **Stand and jump with a hook punch in a circular way.**

Do at least 25 times each hand.

Advanced Medicinal Martial Yoga XXIII) **Lie down on palm with push up position. Hold it for 30secs, without the body touching the ground**

Do it at
least 2 times everyday.

Advanced Medicinal Martial Yoga XXIV **Keep your legs on 2 feet wall.**

Keep your palms on ground.
and hold it for 30 secs.

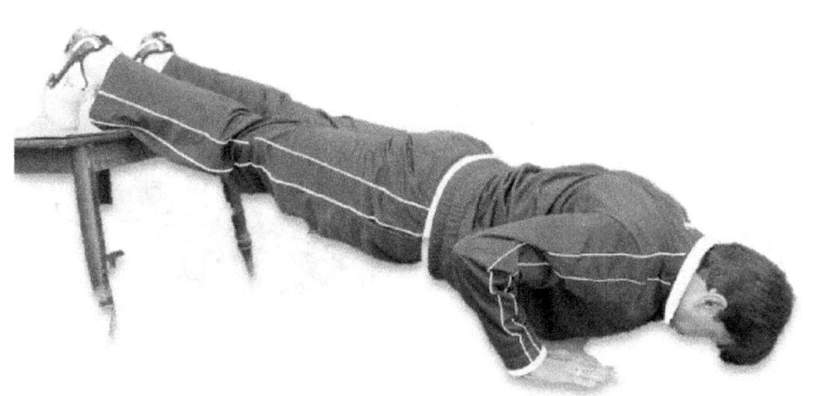

Advanced Medicinal Martial Yoga XXV Lie down with legs at sky level. Rotate your right leg clockwise and anti-clockwise 10 times each. Repeat the same with other leg.
Note: Rotate minimum radius is 2 feet.

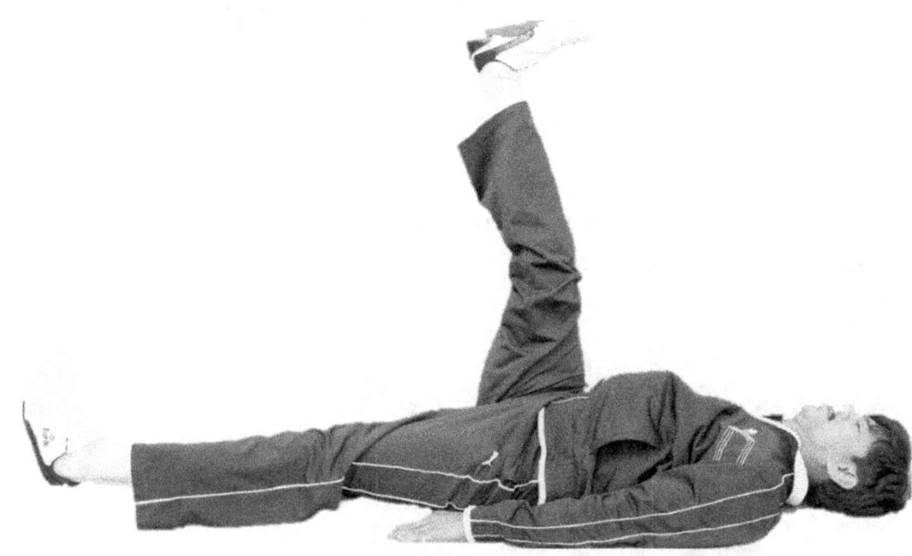

Advanced Medicinal Martial Yoga XXVI) Lie down with legs straight at sky level Split the legs sideways. Do it at least 10 times.

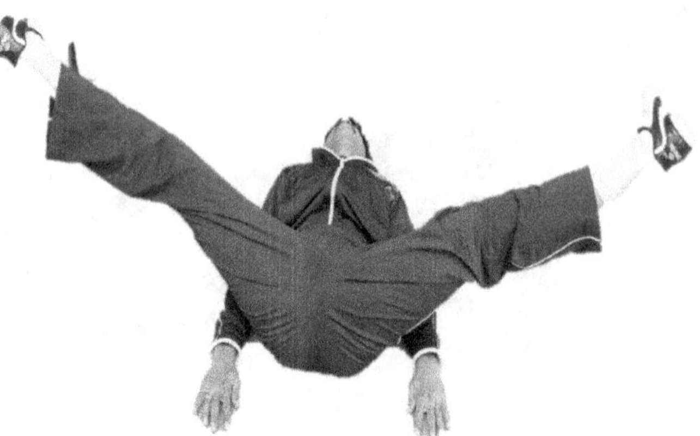

Advanced Medicinal Martial Yoga XXVII) Sit with the knees and hands on thc ground. Kick on the side 10 times each side, without dropping the leg.

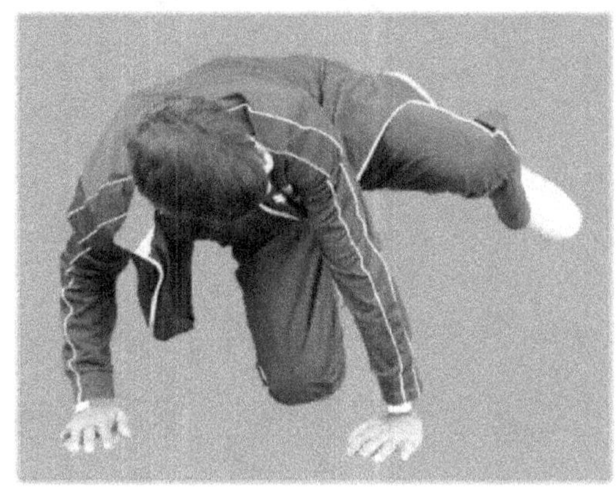

Advanced Medicinal Martial Yoga XXIX) Sit with knees and hands on the ground Kick back side without dropping the legs. Repeat with the other leg. 10   times each leg.

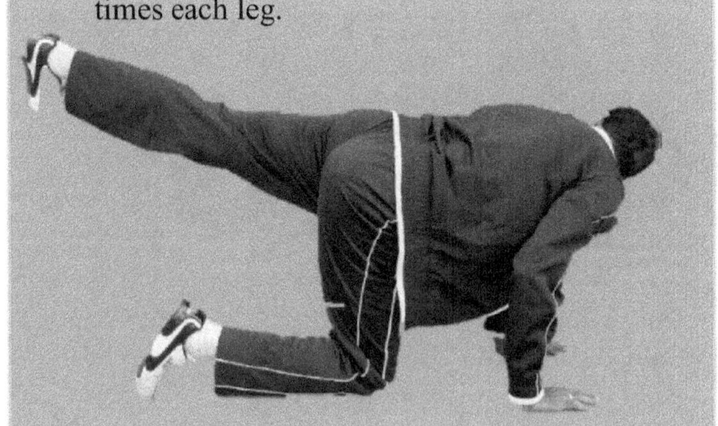

 Horse stance with double the shoulder distance between the legs Hands pressed backwards to maximum. Breath in from abdomen and breath out slowly from
 lower abdomen and Relax !

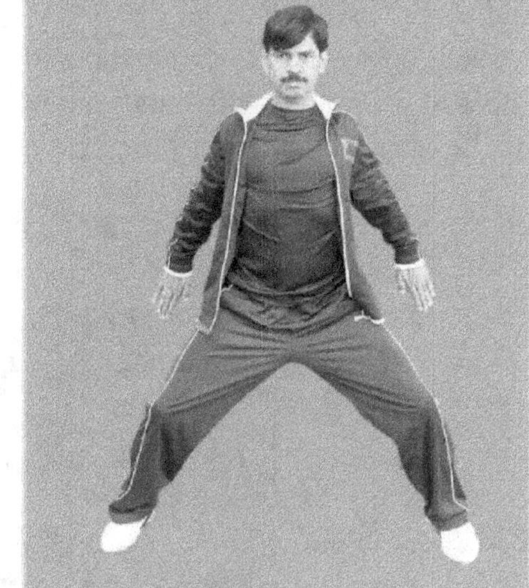

 Lie down sideways with bent knees and split bent knees. Only one leg. Do the same with other side. Do it at least 10 times each side.

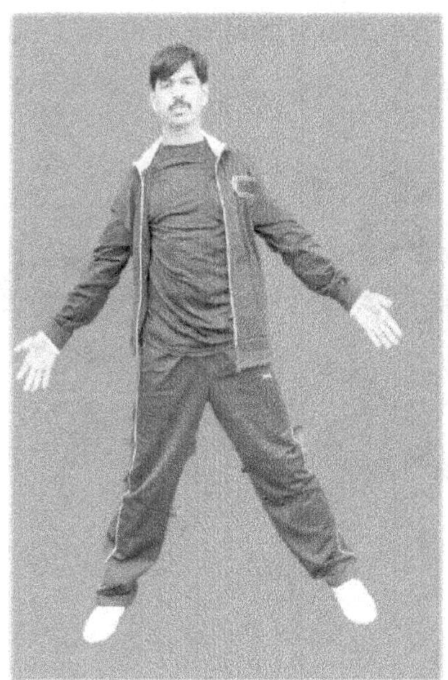

 Horse stance with double the
shoulder distance between the legs. Breath in and bend forwards. Keep your
hands on the navel i.e, left over right hand breath in and control and rotate
the hand harder over the navel
12 times and come back to original position.
Stand up and breath out with hands sideways and do this exercise
for 6 to 12 sets. This is one of the best exercises for internal cleaning.

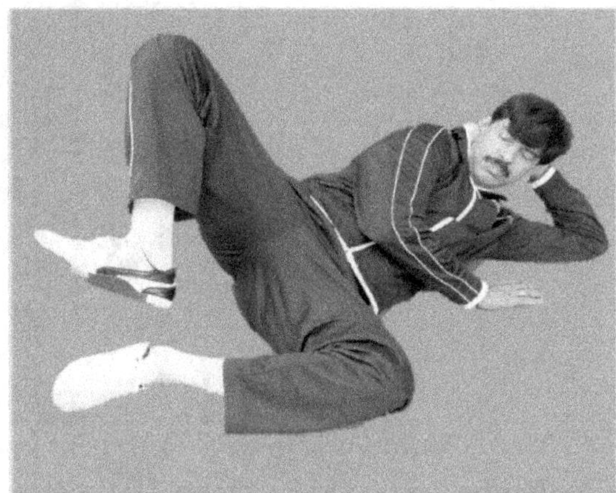

 Here is the list of
most common problems that today's modern human society is facing.

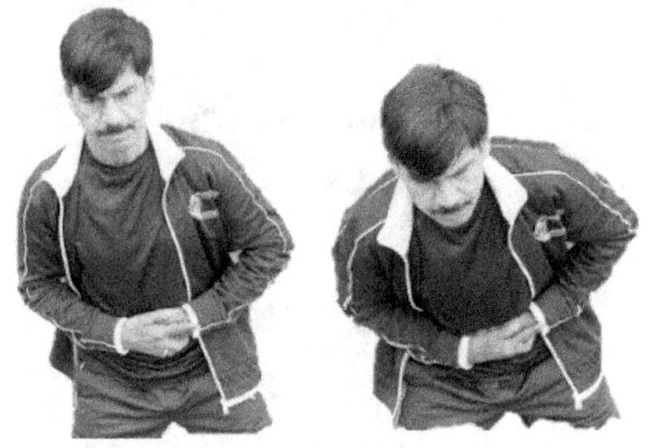

Stress:

Many researchers and physicians around the world are convinced that stress is the main cause of mental illness, cancer, multiple sclerosis, arthritis, peptic ulcers, heart diseases, premature aging, and most importantly blood pressure and diabetics.

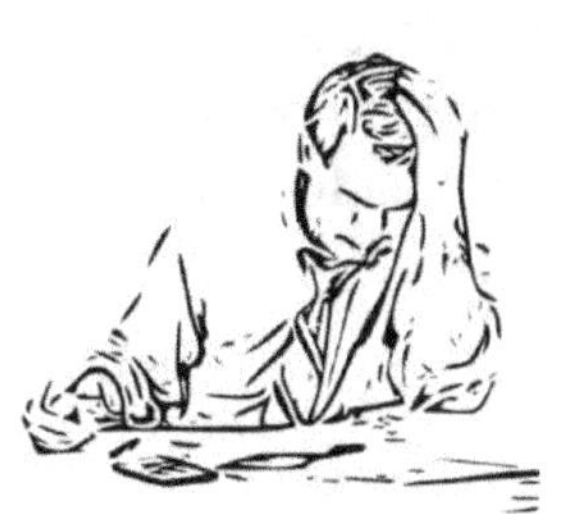

Stress is the prime ailment to cope up in today's world for people of all ages from 10 to 70 years. It is a disgrace that, we humans, are not able to cope up with physical and mental challenges and our bodies become feeble and we lose the excitement of enthusiastic living.

Most of the present world people eat, take bath and brush their teeth daily; but why they forget to clean body organs and muscles with sweating out? Not sweating is the main cause of stress. It is very simple to control stress – with some of the below mentioned strategies

- ✓ Moderation in drinking
- ✓ Adequate sleep
- ✓ Controlling addictions
- ✓ Regular balanced meal
- ✓ Daily physical / medicinal exercises with breathing exercise and organ sounds
- ✓ Proper relaxation

Above mentioned exercises will release many tensions of your day to day life's problems and re-center yourself in yourself with peace with real harmony.

Here we have few extraordinary exercises for a stress-free life

1. Progressive relaxation.
2. Organ healing sounds (six sounds) in the morning.
3. Running for 3 km and after that, keep your legs 3ft inclined, so that more blood flows to head.
4. 8 Brocade exercises – 6 each time.
5. After dinner walk for 1 KM
6. Sit comfortably on easy chair, close your eyes and then count from 100 to 1. If the thoughts come, please try not to go behind the thoughts and continue to count backwards. Once you reach 1, then wait 2 minutes, empty your mind and wake up.
7. Advance technique for mind is take any of your favorite God's names and keep chanting slowly in the mind. Also, count the number of times you are changing. Note: You must do this while seated in a comfortable posture on chair and with eyes closed. Initially you can do for the 50 counts and slowly increase.

Headache and Migraine

Headaches are many types – two side head ache, one sided etc. These headaches

start over straining eyes in the night studies or night duty, long hour jobs as in IT or overstraining physical body or over draining of salt in the body.

Further other problems of over stress of modern world, sleeplessness, worry can also cause headaches. Many are facing issues related to headache/migraine should start physical and mental.

Exercise.

1. Simple Pranayama
2. Walking for 3 kms and keep legs in inclined at 3ft for 3minutes a day, after finishing the walk. This helps to have more blood supply to head.
3. Breathing exercise - Lie down like in Shraavana and breath in from nose and tongue must touch the roof of mount and image the air goes to head and breath out imaging that the air goes from the head to navel. One should do this for 10 minutes – 5 times in the morning and 5 times in the evening.
4. Organ healing sounds – 6 times each sound.
5. Drums of heaven – 1 minute.
6. Massage at the skull edge – 1 minute.
7. Shoulder massage till hand.
8. Thumb pinching or clip hold at thumb or thumb massage – for both thumbs
9. Progressive relaxation.
10. Lied down in Shraavana and keep sand/rice bag of rectangular shape on navel. Breathe in while raising your abdomen and breathe out slowly bringing down the bag at abdomen. Focus your mind on the breath in and out and the weight you are lifting.

Back problems

Back is main part of human body, which separates lower body and

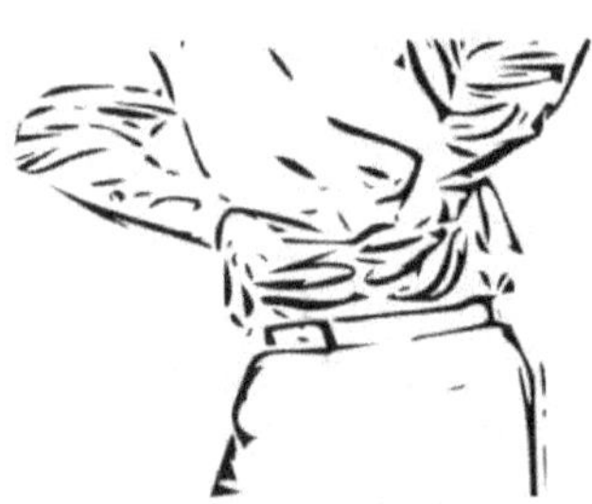

upper body. All the connection muscles, nerves, meridian acupressure points are all inter-connected. So back strengthening is primarily an important activity.
Exercise for back.

1. Massaging lower back with 2 palms of your hand for 1 min daily.
2. Surya namaskars (Sun exercise) 5 times daily.
3. Lie down, spread legs and come up and touch left hand to right leg toes and right hand to left leg toes,10 times each side.
4. Stand and twist back and punch right side and then left side – 10 times each side.
5. Lie down on abdomen with hands sideways and raise your left leg and right leg. Variation- Right hand and right leg straight without bending elbows and knee.
6. Lie down with hand at shoulder level and pull up your hands and legs with each count and come back on ground. See that your upper body and legs including thighs are raised up while doing this exercise.
If your job is to sit long time in the office chair, get up everyone hour from your seat and twist once or twice.

Knee Problems

Knee pain starts with lack of conditioning. Old people stop walking or stop standing for long or do not have enough activity with legs, will attract knee

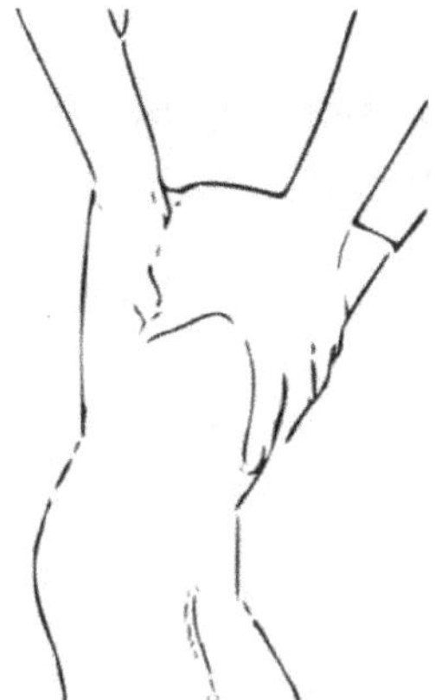

problems. Also, people with diabetic also can catch knee problems. Initially people can get relief from pain by massage or magnetotherapy – by keeping knee magnet continuously for day or two. Then they can start to walk slowly for 1KM. Slowly they can reach 3KMs per day. Next is to start climbing steps around 50 to 100 each day.

Exercise for Knee problems.

1. Stand and hit your back heel to bums (buttocks) left and right legs for 20 times each
2. Walking for 1 to 3 KMs.
3. Climbing steps.
4. One leg forward and other leg backward, bend front leg only and stretch the back leg.
5. Kneel, sit for 10 times every day.
6. Massage knee with your palm by sitting in cross leg position.
7. Use medical knee cap till your knee pain subside.
8. Horse stance (stand with legs stretching with double the shoulder length).
9. Tie the nylon thread to legs and kick front level for 20 each.
10. Jumping on ball of the foot for 20 jumps.

Insomnia/ Sleeplessness

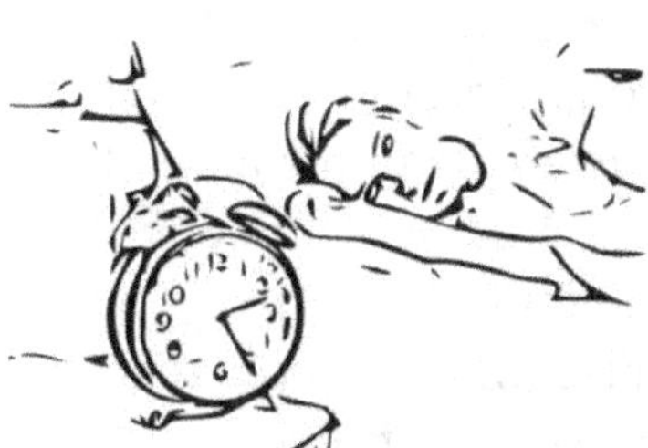

Due to heavy load in head – about business tensions, work load of the job, incomplete studies of students and medical problems of elder people, or any other pending issues of families contribute to the heavy load which is the primary reason for the sleeplessness.

Exercise for Sleeplessness

1. Jogging / Running for 3KMs.
   a. After jogging – Lie down, and keep the legs on 2- or 3-feet table in inclined position, so that blood circulates to the head.
2. All organ healing sounds before going to bed.
3. Eat food 2 hours before you go to sleep.
4. Keep all mobile and other electronic devices in silent mode.
5. Avoid watching Horror movies or sad movies at night.
6. Practice martial yoga.
7. Avoid smoking and heavy drinking liquor/alcohol.
8. Avoid discussing family or business issues at night.

Depression and Anxiety
Exercise suggested for keeping depression and anxiety away.

1. Simple Pranayama.
2. Abdominal breathing.
    a. Lie down on back and keep left hand on navel with pressure. Breathing in slowly and
    b. extend your abdomen and breath out while pulling the abdomen in.
3. 8 brocade exercises.
4. Drums of heaven.

Blood pressure
Exercise suggested for keeping blood pressure under control.

1. Medical exercises – 6 times each.

2. Drum of heaven – 3 minutes.

3. Healing sounds – 6 times each.

4. Martial Yoga.

5. Diet: Avoid Chilies

Diabetes/ Kidney problems
Exercise suggested for keeping kidneys healthy and diabetes under control.

✓ Kidney healing sounds – 24 times daily.
✓ Kidney physical exercises.
✓ Climbing steps – 100 steps every day.
✓ Diet: Avoid eating sweets, rice, banana and custard apple; also avoid salt and sugar.

Obese/Obesity
Today many people from length and breadth of this world is suffering. Obesity is been taken
for granted by people around, even though they know what is best for maintaining a good body.
As you know there are many root causes for hundreds of diseases suffered by our people –

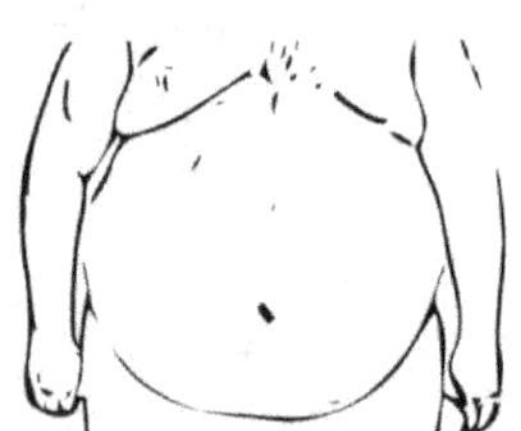

primary reasons are that people do not maintain
a good/healthy diet, no exercise/less exercise. Many people read books
or watch TV programs and follow the obesity reduction schedules by
eating/drinking many powders.
Frankly speaking, the world is lacking knowledge of maintaining the
balanced diet. Thousands of calories they put in every day that are not
able to be burned a day, what happens to the body with these excess calories?

It converts into fat and hence increases the weight of the body – which in turn burdens the knees,
back and burdens every part of physical body. Thereby causing imbalance to the internal body
chemistry and inviting all diseases. The day is not far off where people diet as early as 40 years of
age in this current materialistic world.

I have several of my students who were obese, and they were suffering from thyroid, impotence, heart disease etc., I taught them special exercises to solve obesity.

1. Jogging 5 KMs each day in morning and evening.

2. Martial Yoga.

3. Martial arts training or they can do 1000 punches.

4. Take 2 glasses lime juice with warm water without sugar in the morning.

5. Stop all non-vegetarian food – except Fish.

6. Daily once rice with dal (Lentil) and 2 Chapattis (Flatbread), 2 times a day till he is

    right weight.

7. Abdomen exercise 25 to 50 times – multiple varieties of abdomen exercise.

8. Stand with left hand on navel place right hand (for men) over the left and press hard.

    Breathe in, resist and breathe out while loosening the hands. 10 times a day.

9. Shaping your body size accordingly or reducing weight or sizing of different body

    parts.

    a. If hip size is heavy – bending sideways with hands holding opposite eye and twist

        it to maximum and do it on either side.

In this chapter, I will answer the questions that I got from many of my students, visitors and some eminent personalities. This will surely benefit you.

How will physical fitness help mental health?

Our brains were built for walking—12 miles a day! To improve your brain capacity and thinking, one should move. Physical fitness will ultimately make you fit mentally because all the body receive oxygen internally and externally and thereby makes you feel strong mentally.

Most of the researches confirm that even jog/run of a 3km makes you peaceful and makes you feel stress free. This will keep your angry levels down. Further yoga also tells that breathing exercise helps you mentally free from all mental diseases. There are hundreds of physical exercises which will help you mentally fit.

Exercise: medicinal exercise in this book makes you perfectly fit mentally.

Any tips for waking up early in the morning

Waking up in the morning is not a big task. Many people work late night and sleep, so they require at least 6 to 7 hours of sleep. And one need 1 hour of physical exercise to make your feel refreshed. Further you need to eat dinner with light food, chapattis or fruits and sleep latest 2 hours after your dinner. This will wake you up your desired time. Remember you need at least 6 to 7 hours sleep or else you will have health problems. Take care of sleep.

How can we maintain the same energy levels from morning till night? is there a diet restriction?

Every morning, you need to exercise either martial arts, sports or jogging/running. Add 6 healing organ sounds 6 times each will make you active 24hours of the day.

- Breakfast should be heavy
- Lunch should be 50% of breakfast
- Dinner is only 25% of lunch
- Supper should only be liquid

Exercise: After waking rub your palms each other to produce heat and rub your entire face including ears. Make your face read for 1 minute every day.

How to be focused on the task

When you are advised a task, you should always think whether you have capacity to deal with that task. If it's difficult, you need to take advice from expert. Once the task is assigned to you, you should own it and try with all your energies to complete it. If you need to take help, please do so. Please enjoy doing the task. Every great man on this earth have had task to complete and then only they became famous and known to all of us. Positive thinking always has an advantage for task, project or mission.

Is there any age limit to start Martial arts? What is the minimum and maximum age limits?

Age for doing martial arts is 5 years to 80 years plus. Every moment of martial arts is connected to meridian or acupressure points, even including horse stance position punch with breathing in and out is good for all ages. So is best exercise for 5 to 80 years.

Memory is power house of your mind. You spend 15 mins of your time before you sleep, recall the day's activities in detail with incidents. How the day went, activity you did from getting up to sleep at night It will take 10 to 15 minutes of time. Practice this every day.

Secondly, multiplication exercises. Like multiplying 21x22 =__ Practice this in mind. Keep increasing the complexity of the digits and more. This is very good for memory.

Thirdly, make a habit wherever you go, see things around you and recall immediately.

Fourth: Progressive relaxation. Sit and close your ears and start from head and image every part of your body is relaxing.

E.g., Left toes are relaxing, you must feel that the toes are relaxing and then move on to the next part.

Hair loss is very complicated, but I can tell you one exercise that helps in preventing hair loss. Rub your nails daily 2 minutes in morning (empty stomach) and 2 minutes in the evening.

Second exercise – Stop thinking excessively and stop worrying.

And do lungs healing sound and stomach healing sounds daily 12 times each.

Drinking water is best medicine for all your body. As your body is functioning 24 hours nonstop, till your death – to cool down blood and system in the body, water is a very important ingredient.

Everyone is advised to drink water as frequently as possible. Many researches worldwide advised to drink a glass full of water everyone hour for the age ground of 10 to 100 years. If God hasn't invented water, the entire life on the planet would have died in days.

Ego is against life and not death. Death is the other end of life. In ego they all possess false prestige as if they are supreme and knowledge and feel rich compared to other.

In today's modern world, everyone in one way or other is egoistic. Take egg of a small Child, he always wants to be treated important in the eyes of elders.

Ego is enemy of human civilization and overcoming it is very important and simple too.

Practice to be simple and down to earth. You can't be a leader by commanding people.

When you reflect on the history, all great people who left their legacy are egoless people. They achieved many extraordinary human achievements and are still down to earth. Take my own example. I have achieved several Guinness World Records, but I am very simple, and I associate myself with people of all ages, young and old alike. Ego is considering yourself high and always trying to see the low in others.

Further I can finally say that, people with ego are always at loss and misery. Always behave with courtesy, be thankful to all people – poor, sick, Children, adults and treat everyone The same – junior or senior. Do not differentiate anyone. This is the only secret to overcome ego.

Main reason for stage fear is that people do not have subject knowledge. If they are good in subject, whatever the subject that they are going to speak, then fear never comes. As you know I was having same fear in school and college days. I couldn't realize it then. Now I am an expert in subject matters related to health and longevity, martial arts and universe knowledge. If you ask me to speak on this subject, wherever in the world, I will speak fluently. You must experience the subject knowledge then go on small stage to give a small lecture. You will experience what is lacking, then you will do better every time you face.

I recommend meditation and breathing exercises for helping good public speaking.

They both go hand in hand. Surya namaskars are very good for martial arts and Pranayama as well. The ultimate fitness is only martial arts for age from 5 to 60. Beyond 60, it's only a limited movement advisable. Even in Yoga, beyond 60, people cannot do difficult asanas.

My best advice is martial arts for overall fitness.

Pranayama is the regulation of the breath through certain techniques and exercises.

Press with pressure on eyebrows and edge of eyes for 1 minute.

Looking the nose for 20 seconds and 10 seconds rest; 5 times each.

Massage palms of hands to warm and place them on closed eyes and see blackness through the palm. 30 Seconds.

Sit straight and look at left and right. 5 times.

Sit and rotate eyes clockwise and anticlockwise

Keep left or right index finger in the front of you and concentrate on finger and divert aft3r 5 seconds to other object which is far off (10 to 20 feet away).

Drugs and alcohol are deadly poisons that destroys the brain cells and are cause for nervous disorders including cancer. Initially when people start, as it produces excitement leading to an artificial feeling of self-confident and great strength, people ignore the negative effects of it. Smoking and drinking destroy many organs. Another negative impact of smoking and drinking is, it causes sexual impotence and thereby leading to divorce in many cases. These people think that it's plausible and enjoyable and so the mind gets addicted to it. One must be very careful to associate with people who are addicted to cigarettes or liquor or drugs. Once you taste these, your dependency starts working internally to get rid of pressure of various issues like family, job etc., Lack of fitness leads you more makes these addictions more enjoyable and so you will go with it.

Remember, life is not miserable. It depends on how you use it. Many people do not realize the immense pleasure of your body and life. After reading this whole book of mine, you realize what we are, how we are, and helps plan a better of you – mentally and physically.

Reading is not enough, one must experience. So, please read the book and experience all the exercises for your better tomorrow.

Work is worship. You must work for your family and your Children. This you can't forget. The personal life is different entity and different border where you live with your family. You must balance work and personal life in a very simple way. Don't carry any pending issues or work to other day. Complete the day's work and exit the office. Otherwise, this will lead you to interfere in your personal life and you miss that day. That day long you will keep thinking about not completing the day's work and that spill over to your family time as well.
Do not keep worrying about the task. Keep putting your sincere effort and you will be successful. Do not worry but wait for some time and the work will be done soon. Do not allow your family to interfere it. Keep one task at a time. While you are at work, put all your efforts to complete the work. While you are at home, put your 100% time to the family. Do not mix both.
Life if very shot and we are nearing death faster. Don't worry – be happy.

How to develop good listening skills?

Initially people should take interest in the subject that one likes. Second step is to accept to hear from others, on what they speak about the subject. And what you understand is the most important aspect. If you want to be better than the expert, you need to take interest.
If the subject is of no interest to you, there is no point in in continuing.
E.g., A bed ridden patient cannot hear with any attentiveness if anyone is speaking about Olympic sports. But if he is interested, then he can put his mind.
E.g., If you must talk on a subject, which is of not much interest to audience – you need to link to the audience and how it benefits them. If you and everybody relate to then people will listen.
When you are listening also, you need to first get an idea of the benefit to yourself. Then you're listening skill will improve significantly.

Infertility is the concern among today's newlywed couples.

Couples are facing lot of problem in understanding and coping up with family and relationships. Especially in sexual relationship, these couples are not physically it and hence they are unable to have good relationships. These couples need every day physical.
exercise and develop deep love and intimacy. It needs two persons to know each other in all ways – good and bad, darkness and light. Both should know either side of each other and understand the limitations of each other. Knowing each other is the basic principle of living together – and whatever the problem be, one will support another always.
And the next step to have a happy family is to plan financially. Having a good financial plan is must for happy family life. Poor financial planning led many couples to think of divorce.
In the modern times couples are watching pornographic movies for excitement.
Pornographic/ adult movies are for old people who has lost sexual energy and so they see and enjoy it. They are not for young people. Young people should enjoy subjective and not objective.
History of sex of couples is started way back centuries ago when the couples are unable to have intercourse till orgasm. They started playing foreplay with spouses touching and kissing various places. French discovered that first kissing on the lips is a good starter.

Couples should plan for good and healthy relations. This way couples should start staring their excitement. There are many other reasons one must plan to be very cooperative and understanding. The issues are to be discussed on the table by couples. Otherwise it goes to different direction. Hence more than 50% population is suffering from these misunderstandings.

In Japan islands they lovers and couples rub noses and they think it is perfectly healthy and hygienic. India is also started playing couples with ear lobes and that's perfectly hygienic. This play with ear lobes is very erotic. India discovered the couples playing and kissing ear lobes and there are so many sexual movies, plays and styles and postures which are being enjoyed by the world. In 21st century people are fed-up seeing the same adult style acts, so they started making adult movies with Hollywood actresses and Bollywood actresses and selling with high price to top business and rich people in India and abroad.

Mentak Chia and Maneewan Chiafrom Thailand has made videos and books on cultivating female sexual energy by healing love through the Tao. These couples made healing effect on organs with sexual exercise.

1. Women on top of men with all kisses and touches with tongue etc. will become stimulant and flow of energy to all corresponding organs and has a healing effect.
2. Man, on top of woman will supply energy for woman and solves menstrual problems. Such as cramps and many woman problems.
3. The woman lies on the left side and right leg on man who is opposite facing each other for weakness in bones and joints. Also heals circulation problems.
4. Woman lies on the right side and left on the man who is opposite facing each to her for solving the blood vessel related problems. This also solves the problems related to hardening of the arteries and high blood pressure.
5. Woman lies down with knees bent and man on top will solves the endocrine glands, sexual glands, pancreas and liver. This will also energies general body as a whole.

How to tackle Cholesterol levels and keep heart healthy

Before you eat every time, you should be conscious of what you are going to take in. Conscious of food intake and eating only low cholesterol food, no oily foods, no fatty foods, no red meat at all. Take white meats if you are non-vegetarian. The foremost important is to do exercise and healing sounds for heart and kidneys. Both heart and kidney are interconnected and hence its absolutely needed to do healing sounds for both heart and kidneys. Also, do physical exercises related to heart and kidneys.

Any ergonomic exercises that you suggest for people working at desk for long hours

It is advisable to get up from the chair everyone hour and do few stretches and twisting of fingers, wrist and shoulders. Bend front and back and do all these for 10 seconds. This helps blood circulation. Also, do 2 or 3 deep breaths. These two exercises (stretching and deep breathing) helps you to work for 8 to 12 hours in a day.

Boredom is the enemy to all human beings. You have many things to do in life and where is the time to feel boredom? Boredom is for aged people who finished all societal, family, business obligations and has nothing else think of. There are so many things you can do – meditation, physical exercise.

To maintain a healthy food habit is very difficult in the current Indian scenario as most people are eating junk food on one side and street food on the other side. These foods really damage human body as these foods are made with cheap oil which damage your total health. In India, everyone is busy for simple reason and they prefer to different street food regularly. Further many people start from breakfast to supper eating the outside food. People don't even think what they are eating, how to maintain good health – at least they won't even bother about it. It is a serious matter of concern and we must take care of the health and prevent many diseases. Medical science is a failure in dealing with many diseases. There is no guarantee that we are saved. So, the best thing is to take preventive steps not to get sick. My advices are:
After you wake up and after you are done with brushing, drink one glass of water.

Then go for exercise and then take the breakfast.

From breakfast to lunch, no other food except fruits or liquids/water/juices.

From lunch to dinner, no solid foods to be taken except for water and juices.

You need to maintain these for your good health.

The most important is to make it a point to eat homemade food always. Try spending money on your home food and avoid junk foods. This is your body – God's gift – and you must take care of it. Whenever possible, take seasonal food and eat in empty stomach. Try not to drink water immediately after eating food. Drink half an hour before food or one or two hours after eating food. Whole world must think what they are puffing in the stomach – which will directly impact your health and longevity.

People, if they are happy – they do not think of health, they go busy with their business and education, job etc. When they have headache, then they think as to why it has come? Same with any sickness. People only think only when body faces a problem. This should not be the case. You need to think every day about the body and health, whether you are healthy or sick. You must plan a time for exercises to make complete body fit. Disease is not going to tell you – beware, I am going to come and then you can start reacting to it. In America, people after 40 years age go for health checkups every year. It is a must. In India, people think it is a strange thing, and when I do not have any sickness – why should I have to visit hospital for checkup. We must monitor our health and the most priceless life. You cannot buy life. The whole world is very ignorant, and they never take care life but take care of property, business, job and family. If one takes care of health proactively, 99% of today's diseases won't even exist in our body. Diseases will be born in our body and not outside.

Disease won't come from nature. Diseases are the result of improper care for the body. There are simple ways to create a healthy plan for your body, mentioned in the book.

What is relaxation? How to be relax? Do I need to achieve something to able to lead a relaxed life? There is no need to achieve anything in life to be relaxed. Relaxation means – not the past and not even the future. It's just living in now and enjoying the present moment. Many people serving sentence in jails are peaceless. The main reason is that they think, how it happened, what happens next, why is my fate like this etc. But everything is already over. Whatever crime and theft being done is over and your duty is over, and the government duty too. No need to think much. Be relaxed. Don't burn the candle from both ends. One end is the crime that was already committed. The other end is – worry. Relax. I heard when Dionysus asked Alexander, what are you going to do when you conquer the whole world? Alexander replied – I think, I will relax. Dionysus asked, is it a condition that you should conquer the world to be relaxed? And Dionysus told, how am I relaxed? In many occasions, Alexander said that I never forget the message my whole life. What the man has said was right. There is no condition. If you want to relax you can relax now. You need not postpone it, even for a single moment, because relaxation needs no pre-condition. All it needs is for you to want to relax….

that's it. Relax.

Present world's mind gets involved in many reasons in search of relaxation
-how, methods, techniques, strategies and the whole idea of relaxation is forgotten. Then you are again in a trip of finding methods and those are thousands of masters spoil your mind by teaching many confused methods to relax. My experience is to do best is progressive relaxation with healing sounds and breathing exercises.

Thank you!

I thank brothers, Mr. M. Krishna Reddy and Mr. Sridhar Reddy, who inspired me to seek the wisdom of health, wellness and longevity for the benefit of the whole world.

Many thanks to Anil Kumar Vuchi and his family for typing, designing and setting the pictures and thanks to VVS Prasad for taking the action pictures.

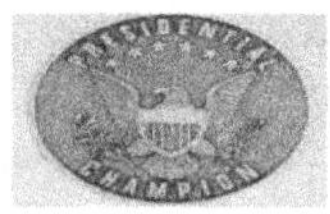 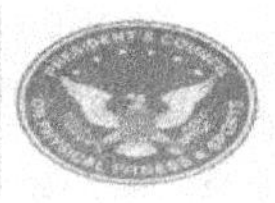 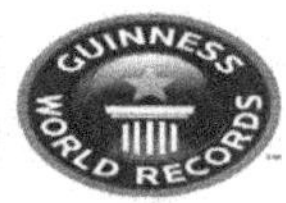 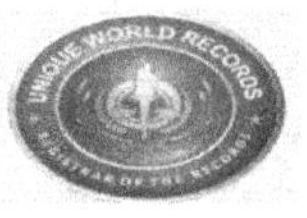 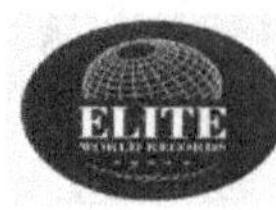 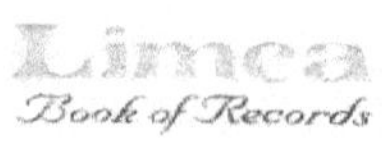

M. JAYANTH REDDY www.mjayanthreddy.com

mjayanthreddy03@gmail.com

Cell : +91 9246829596, 9391007598

Grand master Jayanth Reddy has made himself as well as India proud through this triumph by accomplishing 29 Guinness World Records, Asian Records, 12 American Presidential Awards, multiple Indian Awards, In the Field of Martial Arts and Fitness, "A path on which no Indian has ever treaded before".

Educational Qualification

Doctorate	: Ph.D. in 1992 from American Martial Art University, USA
Post-Graduation	: M.Sc., (Sports Medicine), University of Revenhurst, Netherland.
Graduation	: BSc.,
Diploma	: Dip. In acupressure & Magnet Therapy, Bombay – 1988
	: Dip. In Alternative Therapies, Hyderabad – 1989

Courses Qualified

- Psyche Pranic Healing – Under Institute of Inner Studies, Philippines
- Hypnosis & Self Hypnosis under 'Hypnotic Centre India', T.M. & Siddhi Programme & Yoga under Institute of Maharishi Mahesh Yogi – 1986
- Self-Hypnosis under 'SKYLVIA ACKERMAN', New York, USA in 1986
- CHI POWER Meditation under S.P.C., USA in 1991
- Advance course in QI Gong under Master Mantak CHINA, USA
  Advance course in Taekwondo under various Grand Masters all over the world

Achievements in Taekwondo (National & International)

29 Times Guinness World Record holder.

- 'Fastest Puncher' in the world! Broke the previous Guinness and Olympic record.

- Holds the world record for Maximum number of kicks in one hour wearing 10 Kgs of ankle weights.

- 8th Dan in Taekwondo.

- Conferred Highest DAN by World Taekwondo Masters Association.

- Won Gold Medal in British Open International Taekwondo Championship in 2002 – England.

- Won Bronze Medal in World Taekwondo Championship in Oct' 1988 – England.

- Won Bronze Medal in British International Taekwondo Championship in Oct' 1999 – London.

- Won 5 Gold Medals in Nationals including National Games.

- Won Silver Medal in National Games Taekwondo Championship in New Delhi – 1985.
- **Black Belt V Dan:** World Taekwondo Chang Moo Kwan Federation – Seoul, Korea.

- **Black Belt V Dan:** United Nations Martial Arts Federation, New York.

- **Black Belt VI Dan:** World Martial Arts Masters Federations, U.S.A.

- **Black Belt VIII Dan:** World Taekwondo Jidokwan, Korea – 2010.

Award Winner & Honors (National & International)

- Presidential Champion Award – **Gold Award** – Mar' 2005.
- Graduation Certificate award in International Poomsae Referee Seminar , Dubai , U.A.E , Jul' 2004.
- **Citation** award from the **WTF President,** Korea – 2003.
- Presidential Active Life Style award by **George W. Bush** in Aug' 2002.
- Presidential Physical Fitness award by **George W. Bush** in Aug' 2002.
- National Physical Fitness award by **George W. Bush** in Aug' 2002.
- **International Hall of Fame** in 1999 – USA.
- Presidential Sports Award by **George Bush & Bill Clinton** in 1998 & 1991.
- Cyprus run for **Humanity in the cause of AIDS & Physical Fitness Awareness** -2008.
- Presidential Champion Award from Barack Obama, President of United States –10th December 2010.
- Guinness World Record 2010 in Taekwondo – August 2010.
- Guinness World Record 2011 in Taekwondo – April- 2011.
- Physical Fitness Award – August 2010.
- Participated as a coach in Asian Gold Cup Taekwondo Championship – 2007 in Hongkong & Open. Taekwondo Championship – 2010.

- Appreciation award for Promoting Taekwondo Martial Arts in India from **Kang Won-Sik,** President of Kukkiwon, Korea on 11th December 2010.

Personal Profile
- Date of Birth   :   :14th December
- Founder & President   :JR International Taekwondo Academy (India)
- Founder   :Andhra Pradesh Taekwondo Association
- President   :Hyderabad District Taekwondo Association
- Chairman   :INFINIO Tae Kwond Do World

- Former Joint Secretary   :Taekwondo Federation of India
- Tech. Committee Member   :Former Taekwondo Federation of India
- Graduate   :In Poomsee (WTF)
- Organizer   :As an organizer conducted State /
  National Championships & Federation
- Vice-Chairman   :Running for Humanity Cyprus Run for AIDS Awareness
  and Physical Fitness.
- Managing Partner   :Morramganti Construction, Hyderabad.
-
-

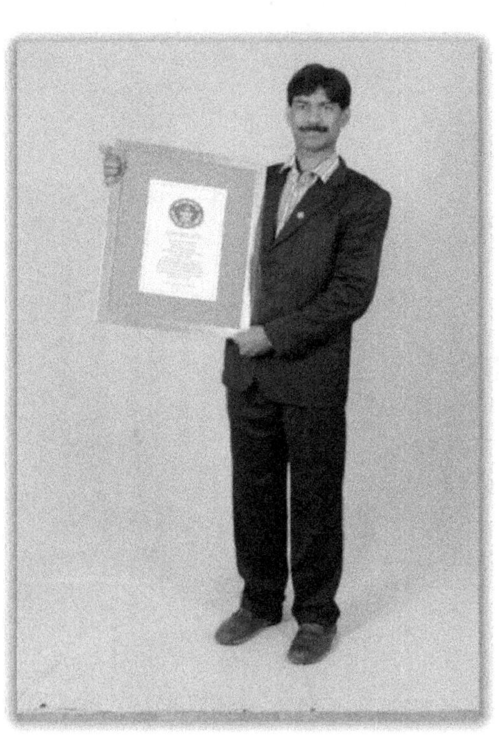

Grand Master M. Jayanth Reddy is a Highest DAN in Taekwondo and holds 28 Guinness World Records along with 34 other world records. You can know more about him at www.mjayanthreddy.com

This is a gift to humanity from the great grand master. This book primarily incorporates all the knowledge that Mr. Jayanth Reddy acquired over years from various other masters, martial art techniques and his travels across the length and breadth of the globe.

You can find multiple techniques and tips to keep healthy and live a minimum of 100 years with ease and no to 'Disease'.